BEGINNER AERIAL SILKS POSE GUIDE

STATIC TRICKS FOR THOSE LOOKING TO DIVE INTO THE WORLD OF AERIAL SILKS

BY: SAM MELLOR

PHOTOS: JENYA KUSHNIR

MODEL: MARINA TURNER

ALL RIGHTS RESERVED.
NO PART OF THIS PUBLICATION MAY BE REPRODUCED, STORED IN A RETRIEVAL SYSTEM, OR TRANSMITTED IN ANY WAY OR BY ANY MEANS, ELECTRONIC, MECHANICAL, PHOTOCOPYING, RECORDING OR OTHERWISE, WITHOUT THE PRIOR WRITTEN PERMISSION OF SAM MELLOR.

IT IS RECOMMENDED THAT YOU CHECK WITH YOUR DOCTOR OR HEALTHCARE PROVIDER BEFORE BEGINNING NEW EXERCISE PROGRAMS.

WHILST EVERY CARE HAS BEEN TAKEN IN THE PREPARATION OF THIS MATERIAL, THERE IS A REAL CHANCE OF INJURY IN EXECUTION OF THE MOVEMENTS DESCRIBED IN THIS BOOK. THE PUBLISHERS AND ALL PERSONS INVOLVED IN THE MAKING OF THIS MANUAL WILL NOT ACCEPT RESPONSIBILITY FOR INJURY TO ANY DEGREE, INCLUDING DEATH, TO ANY PERSON AS A RESULT OF PARTICIPATION IN THE ACTIVITIES DESCRIBED IN THIS MANUAL. PURCHASE OR USE OF THIS DOCUMENT CONSTITUTES AGREEMENT TO THIS EFFECT. FURTHERMORE, RIGGING OF AERIAL EQUIPMENT IS NOT DISCUSSED IN THIS MANUAL. CONSULT A PROFESSIONAL RIGGER WHEN IT COMES TO USING ANY HANGING EQUIPMENT.

PUBLISHED BY: CREATESPACE.COM

UNITED STATES OF AMERICA

ISBN-13:
978-1515309826

ISBN-10:
1515309827

FORWARD

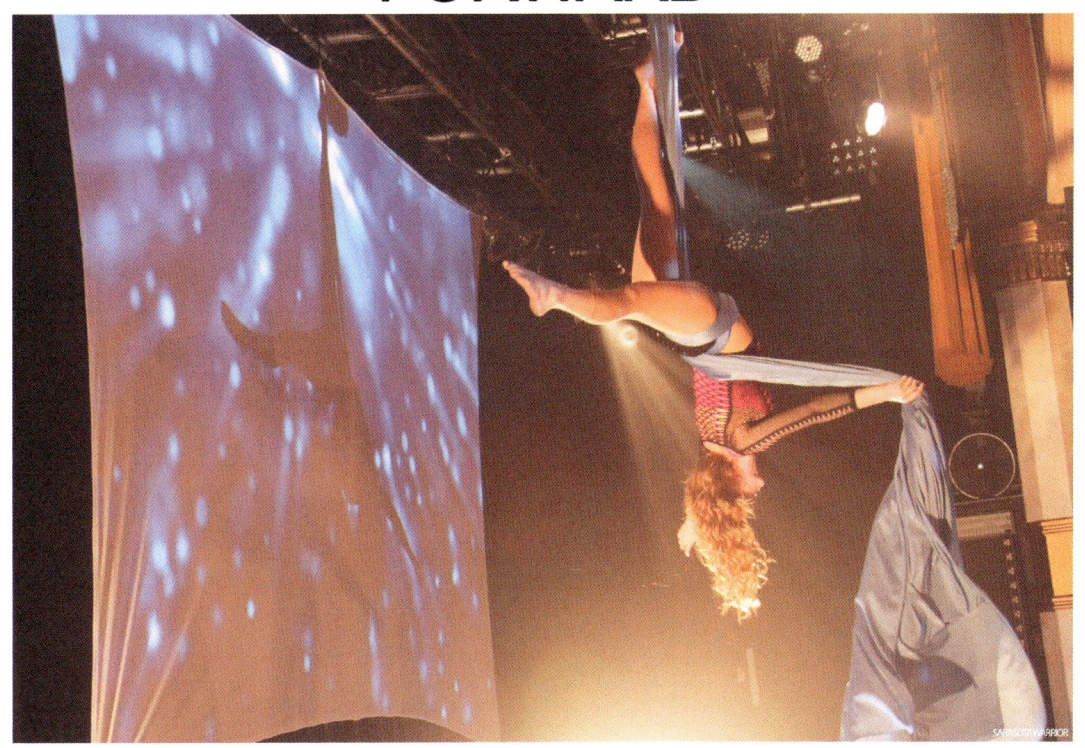

Thank you so much for purchasing this manual!

This has been an absolute delight to put together and I'm very excited to share it with you. Aerial silks has been my passion for a number of years now and I hope it becomes yours aswell. If you come across anything in this manual that stumbles / confuses you please feel free to contact me through any of my social media sites!

The world of aerial silks is quite vast and much can be left up to the imagination when it comes to performing tricks, creating poses and growing with this art. The poses listed in this guide are just a few of my favorite beginner poses. As you learn these, listen to your body and feel free to get creative. In the back of this book you'll find illustrations of variations of the poses covered. Many of these were discovered through students listening to their body and exploring the fabric.

With that in mind, injury is still a very real possibility in an art likethis so practice with awareness and care.

Care for your rigging and your fabric! Your fabric should be quality fabric and tested / designed to be load bearing. Be mindful of your rigging, make sure it is secure and again designed for load bearing. It is recommended to hire a professional rigger and to practice with mats underneath you.

Be aware of your body and your strength. I have seen many people (myself included) injure themselves due to improper or no warm up / stretching. It is very important to warm up before practicing this art. The fabric can force the body in directions you are not used to and gravity can cause you to drop heavily into a position you're not prepared for.

Reserving your strength is something else you should keep in mind while practicing. It's easy to forget that you need just as much strength to get into the pose as well as out of the pose. Always master the entry and exit of the trick low before taking it higher. When in doubt , have a buddy / spotter there for you!

Silks can be trying but yet very rewarding so stick with it and stay safe!

I hope you have a blessed silk journey!

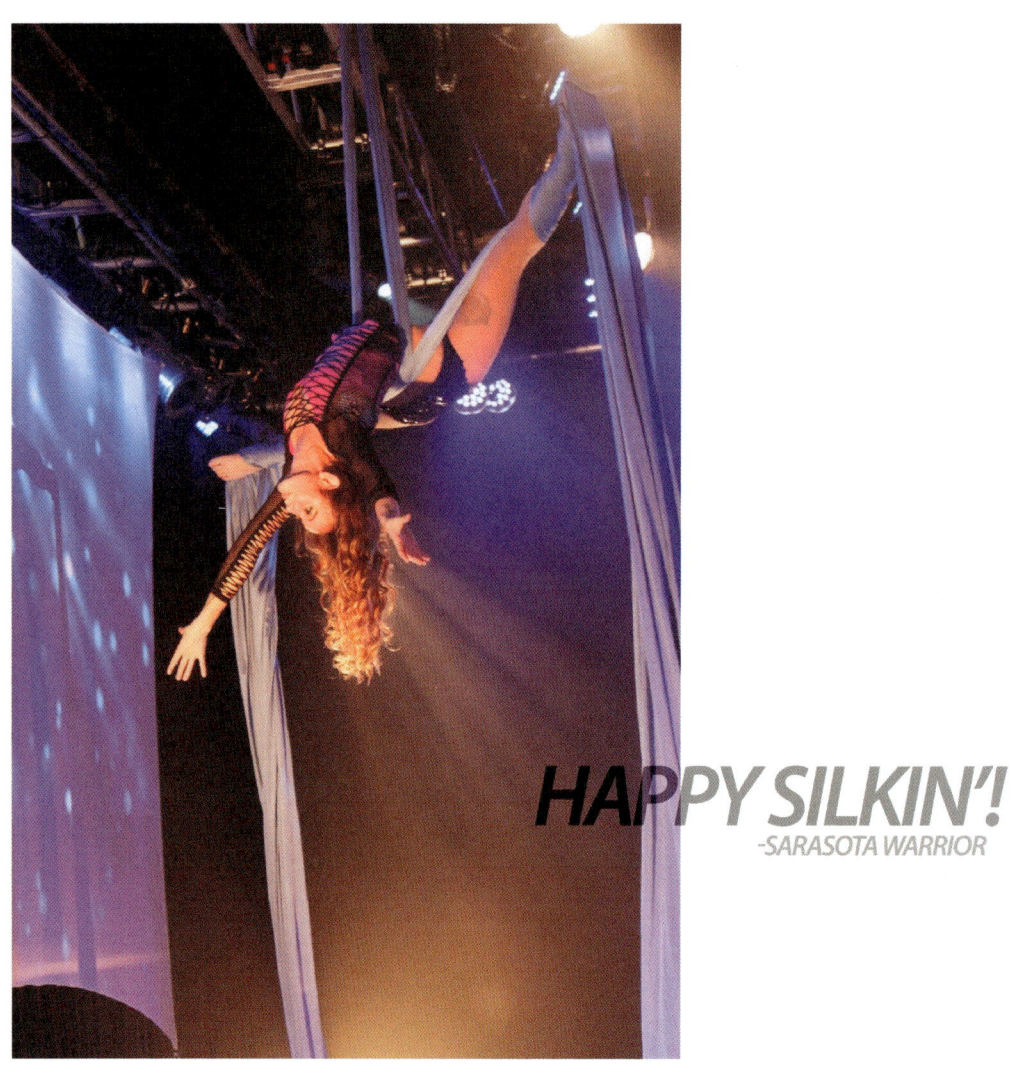

HAPPY SILKIN'!
-SARASOTA WARRIOR

FACEBOOK: SARASOTA WARRIOR

INSTAGRAM: @SARASOTAWARRIORSTUDIO

EMAIL: INFO@SARASOTAWARRIOR.COM

WWW.SARASOTAWARRIOR.COM

TABLE OF CONTENTS

CHAPTER 1 - KEY TERMS AND WARM UP - PG 1

KEY TERMS - PG 2, 3
WARM UP - PG 4, 5, 6, 7

CHAPTER 2 - SINGLE AND DOUBLE FOOTLOCKS - PG 8

DANCER USING HANDS - PG 9
DANCER WITHOUT USING HANDS - PG 10
FIGURE 8 USING HANDS - PG 11
FIGURE 8 WITHOUT USING HANDS - PG 12
DOUBLE FOOTLOCK USING HANDS - PG 13
DOUBLE FOOTLOCKS WITHOUT USING HANDS - PG 14

CHAPTER 3 - WRIST WRAP POSES - PG 15

WRIST WRAP - PG 16
BASIC POSES - PG 17, 18
BIRDS NEST - PG 19
SPLIT THROUGH - PG 20
PIGEON - PG 21

CHAPTER 4 - SINGLE FOOTLOCK POSES - PG 22

LADYSIT - PG 23
DRAMA QUEEN AND ATTITUDE - PG 24
TURNOUT - PG 25
STAR TURNOUT - PG 26
SHOULDER DROP THROUGHS - PG 27
FORWARD PENDULUM - PG 28
REVERSE PENDULUM - PG 29
DANCER - PG 30
BOW AND ARROW - PG 31

MERMAID - *PG 32, 33*
LIBERTY LEAN - *PG 34*
COCOON - *PG 35*
MAN IN THE MOON - *PG 36*
CLOTHESLINE - *PG 37*
360 TWIST - *PG 38, 39*
MARIONETTE - *PG 40, 41*
MARIONETTE INTO DANCER - *PG 42*
FLAG - *PG 43, 44*
LADYSIT HANG - *PG 45*
LOTUS HANG - *PG 46*

CHAPTER 5 - DOUBLE FOOTLOCK POSES - *PG 47*

SPLITS - *PG 47*
SPLIT ROLL UP - *PG 48, 49*
CUPID SEAT - *PG 50, 51*
CROSSBACK STRADDLE - *PG 52, 53*
SPIDERMAN - *PG 54*
BUDDHA - *PG 55*

CHAPTER 6 INVERSIONS - *PG 56*

INSIDE LEG HANG - *PG 57*
ANGEL - *PG 58*
ANGEL EXIT - *PG 59*
SCORPION - *PG 60*
CRUCIFIX WRAP - *PG 61*
CRUCIFIX PIGEON - *PG 62*

CHAPTER 7 - CONDITIONING EXERCISES - *PG 63*
BASIC EXERCISES - *PG 63, 64*

CHAPTER 8 - INSPIRATIONAL POSES - *PG 65*

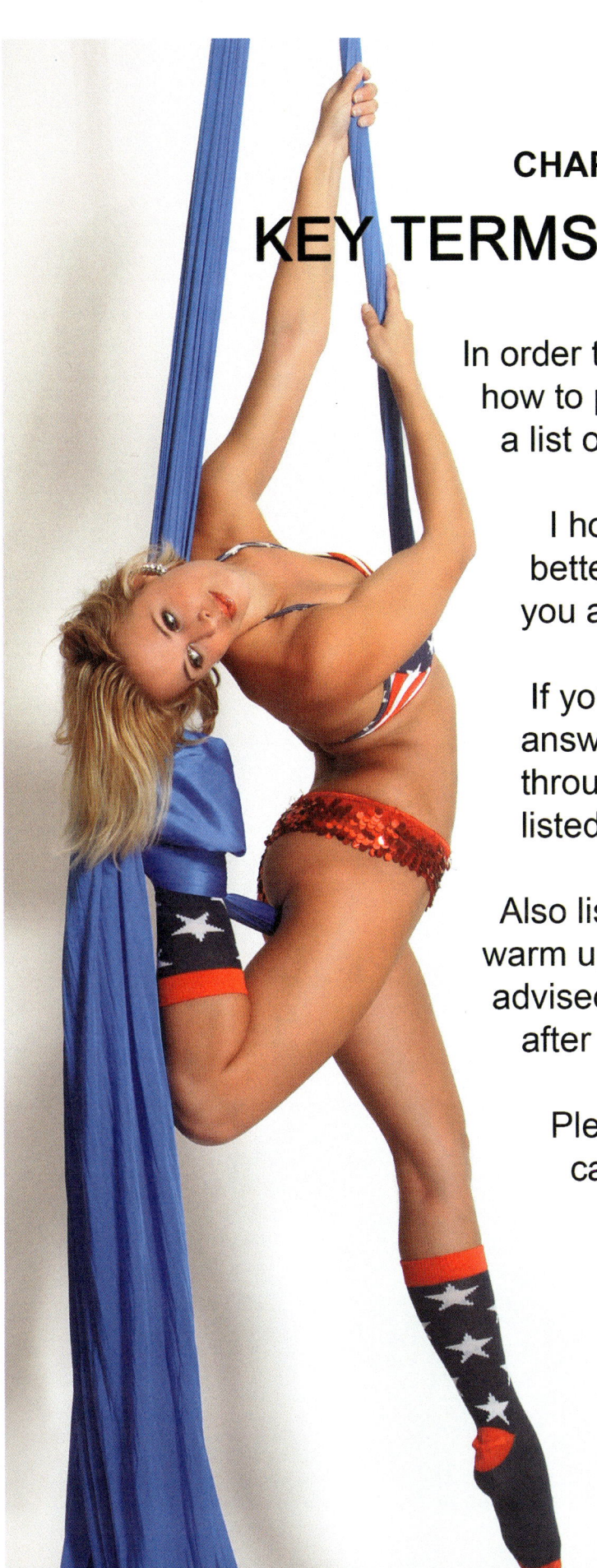

CHAPTER 1
KEY TERMS AND WARM UP

In order to successfully understand how to perform these poses i've created a list of key terms . . .

I hope these terms will help you better understand the moves while you are practicing.

If you have any confusion I am open to answering questions / concerns through any of my social media sites listed in my foreward! :)

Also listed in this chapter are a few warm up stretches that are strongly advised for you to perform before / after each practice.

Please remember to practice with care and intelligience! ! !

INSIDE ARM
THE ARM CLOSEST TO THE FABRIC

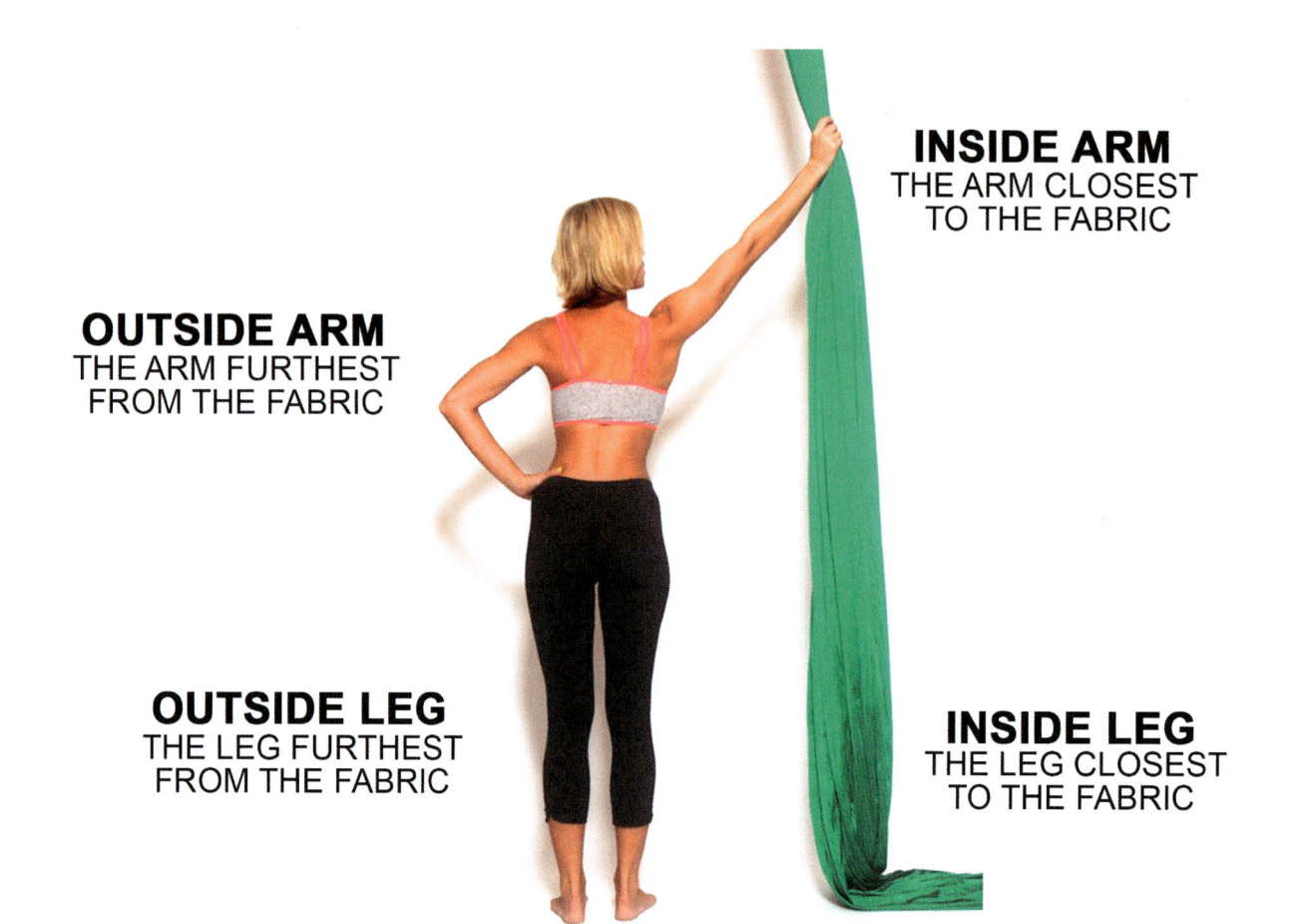

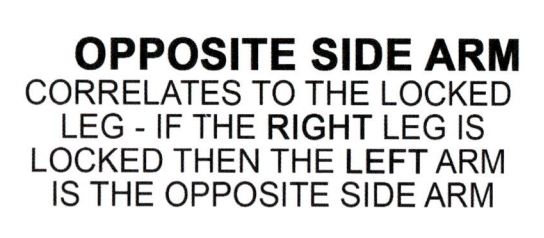

OUTSIDE ARM
THE ARM FURTHEST FROM THE FABRIC

OUTSIDE LEG
THE LEG FURTHEST FROM THE FABRIC

INSIDE LEG
THE LEG CLOSEST TO THE FABRIC

SAME SIDE ARM
CORRELATES TO THE LOCKED LEG - IF THE **RIGHT** LEG IS LOCKED THEN THE **RIGHT** ARM IS THE SAME SIDE ARM

OPPOSITE SIDE ARM
CORRELATES TO THE LOCKED LEG - IF THE **RIGHT** LEG IS LOCKED THEN THE **LEFT** ARM IS THE OPPOSITE SIDE ARM

FREE LEG
THE LEG THAT IS NOT IN A FOOTLOCK

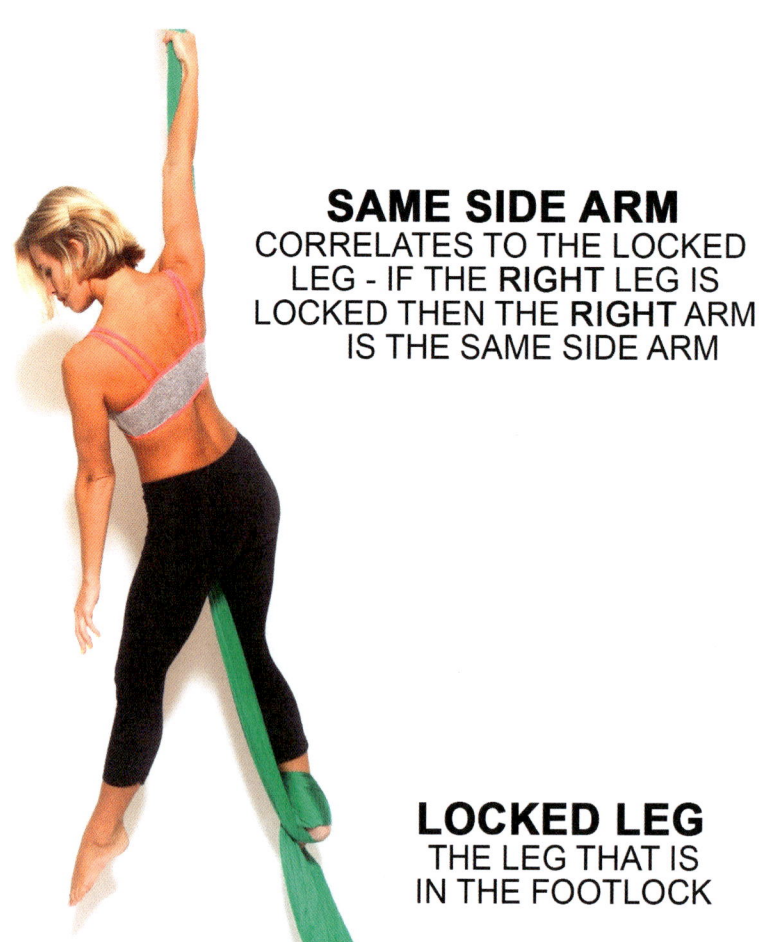

LOCKED LEG
THE LEG THAT IS IN THE FOOTLOCK

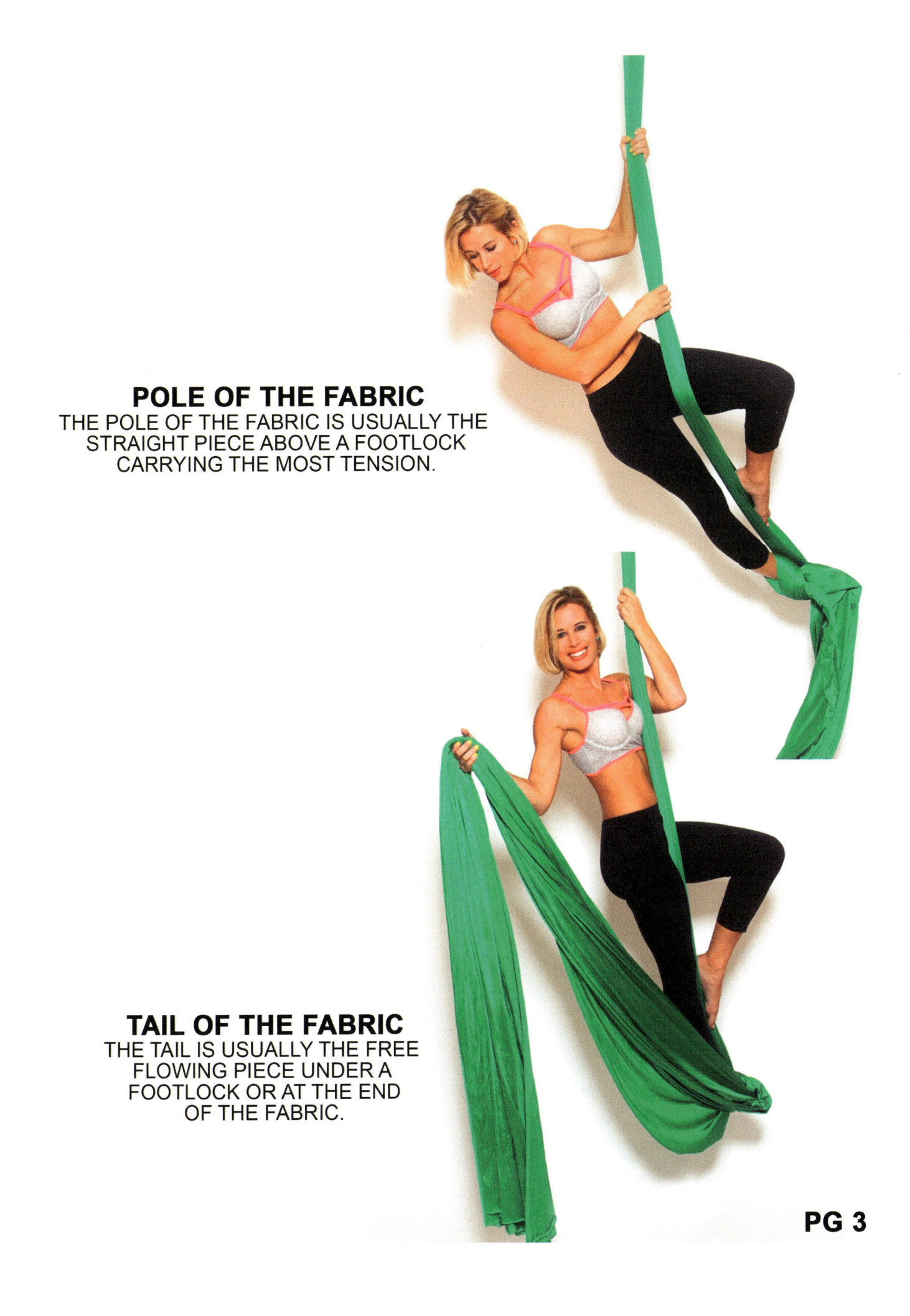

POLE OF THE FABRIC
THE POLE OF THE FABRIC IS USUALLY THE STRAIGHT PIECE ABOVE A FOOTLOCK CARRYING THE MOST TENSION.

TAIL OF THE FABRIC
THE TAIL IS USUALLY THE FREE FLOWING PIECE UNDER A FOOTLOCK OR AT THE END OF THE FABRIC.

WARM UP STRETCHES
"BETTER TO SPEND 10 MINUTES STRETCHING THEN 10 DAYS INJURED!"

Here are a few simple stretches you can do before and after your practice. . . Keep in mind stretching is extemely beneficial and can save you from many unecessary injuries.

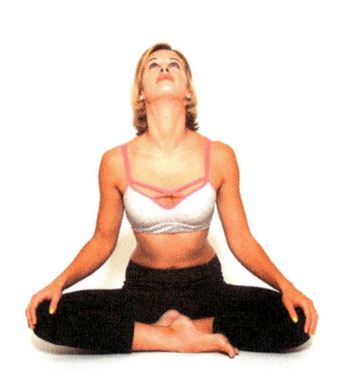

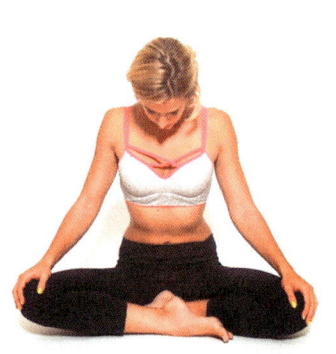

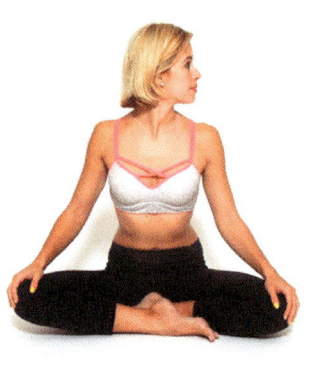

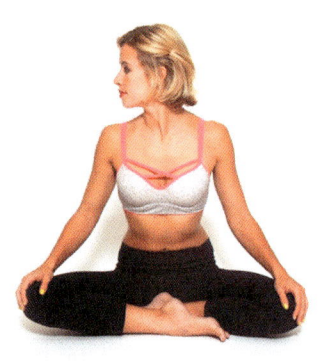

NECK STRETCHES: DOWN , UP , SIDE TO SIDE

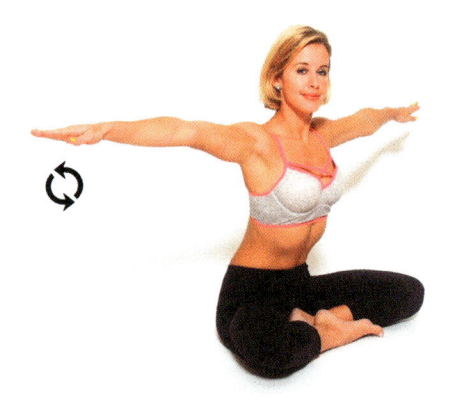

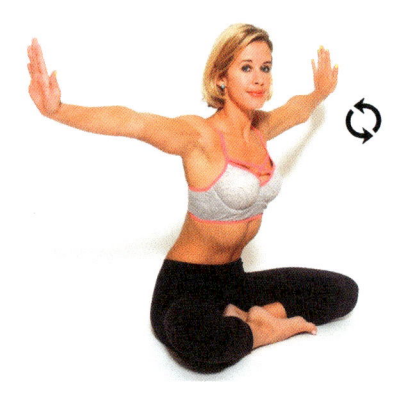

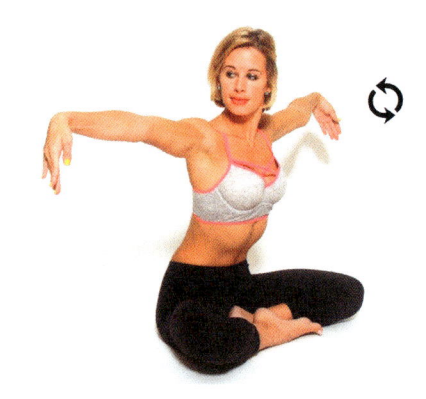

FORWARD AND REVERSE SHOULDER CIRCLES
1. PALMS STRAIGHT 2. PALMS UP 3. PALMS DOWN

Circles are one of my favorite ways to prepare the shoulders for practice . . . Do about 20 in each direction and you will be nice and warm! This is also a great way to tone those glorious flappy 'wings' we all love under the biceps! ;)

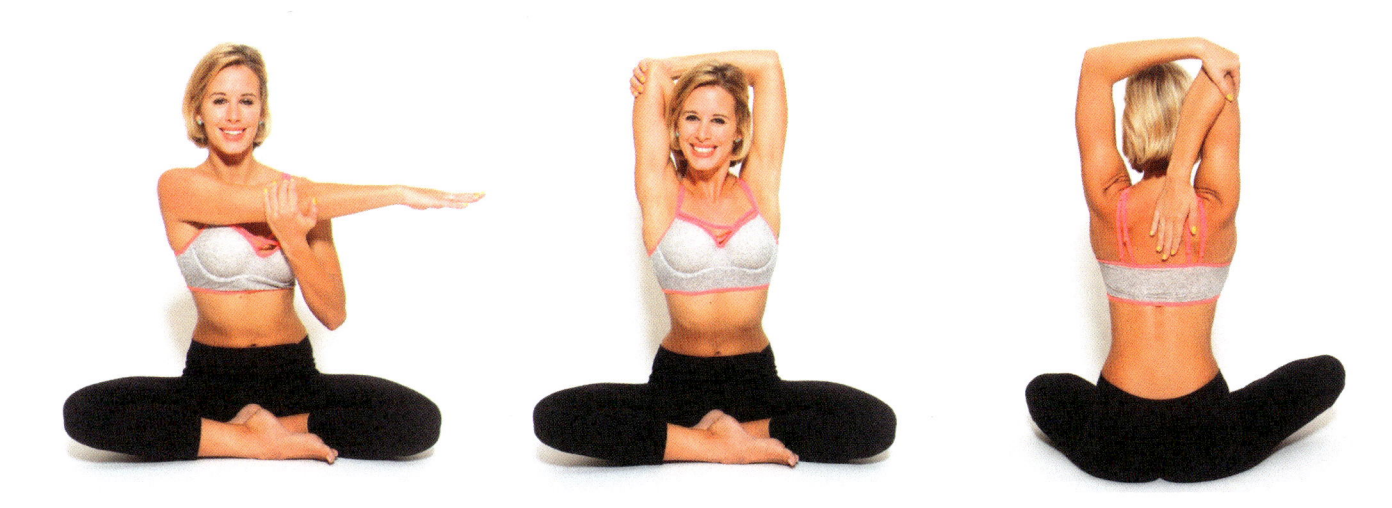

Arm across the chest - be sure to keep your palm at least shoulder level.

Arm behind the head - imagine your trying to pat yourself on the back. pull the elbow as far behind the head as your can.

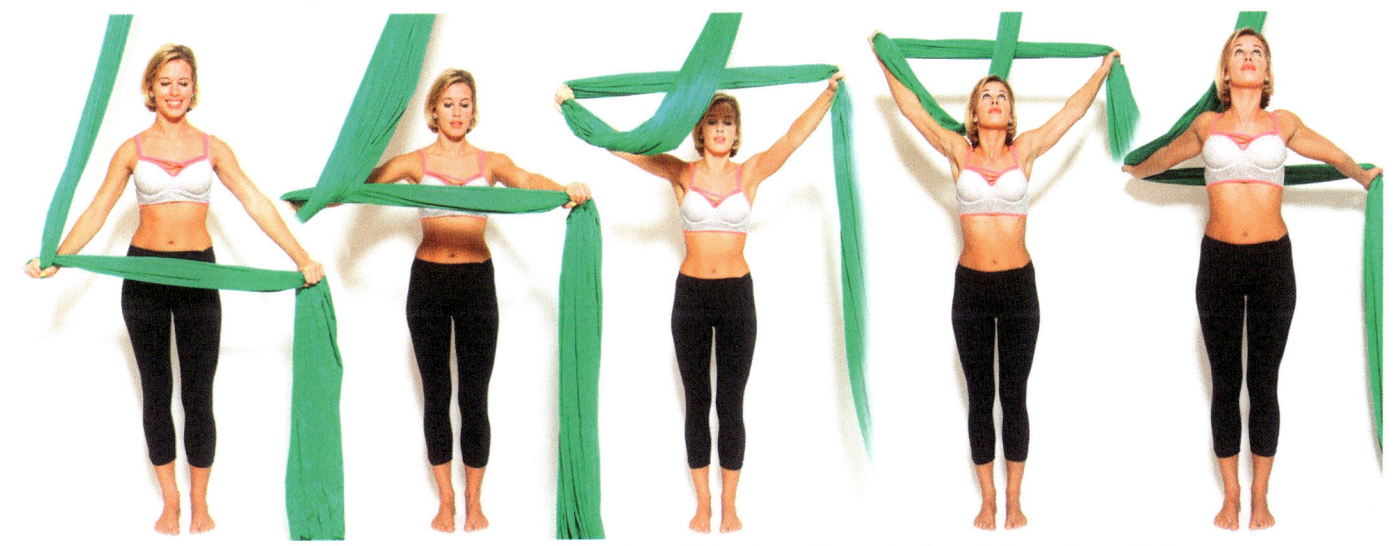

Shoulder joint rotation - grip the fabric about double shoulder width apart. rotate the fabric back and forth from front to back.

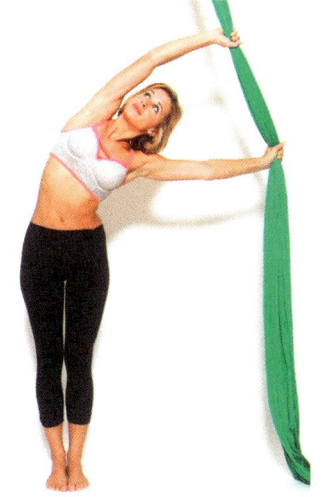

Standing side stretch - stand with your feet side by side , grip the fabric above the head and reach over . . . keep an even amount of weight distributed between both feet.

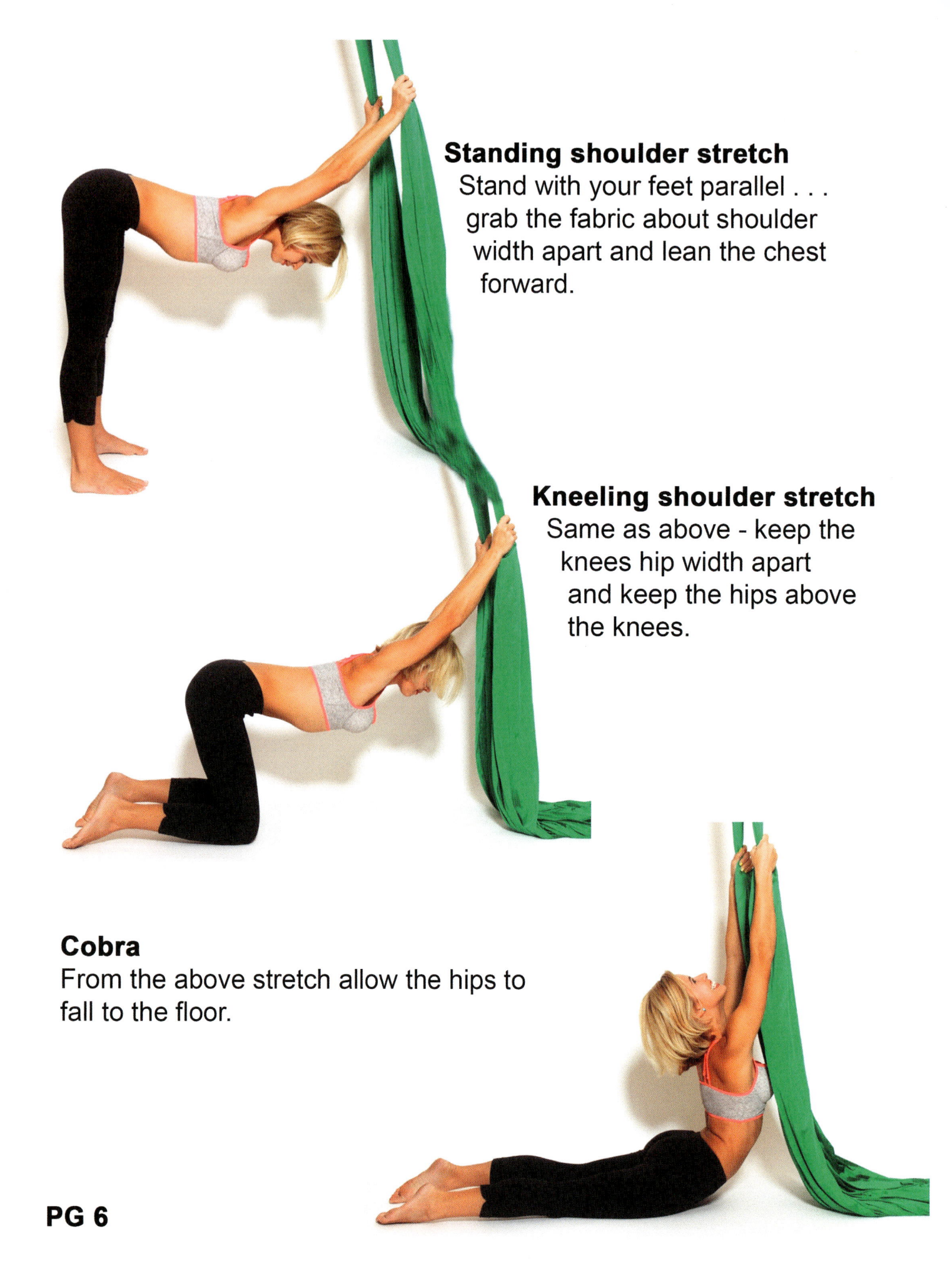

Standing shoulder stretch
Stand with your feet parallel . . . grab the fabric about shoulder width apart and lean the chest forward.

Kneeling shoulder stretch
Same as above - keep the knees hip width apart and keep the hips above the knees.

Cobra
From the above stretch allow the hips to fall to the floor.

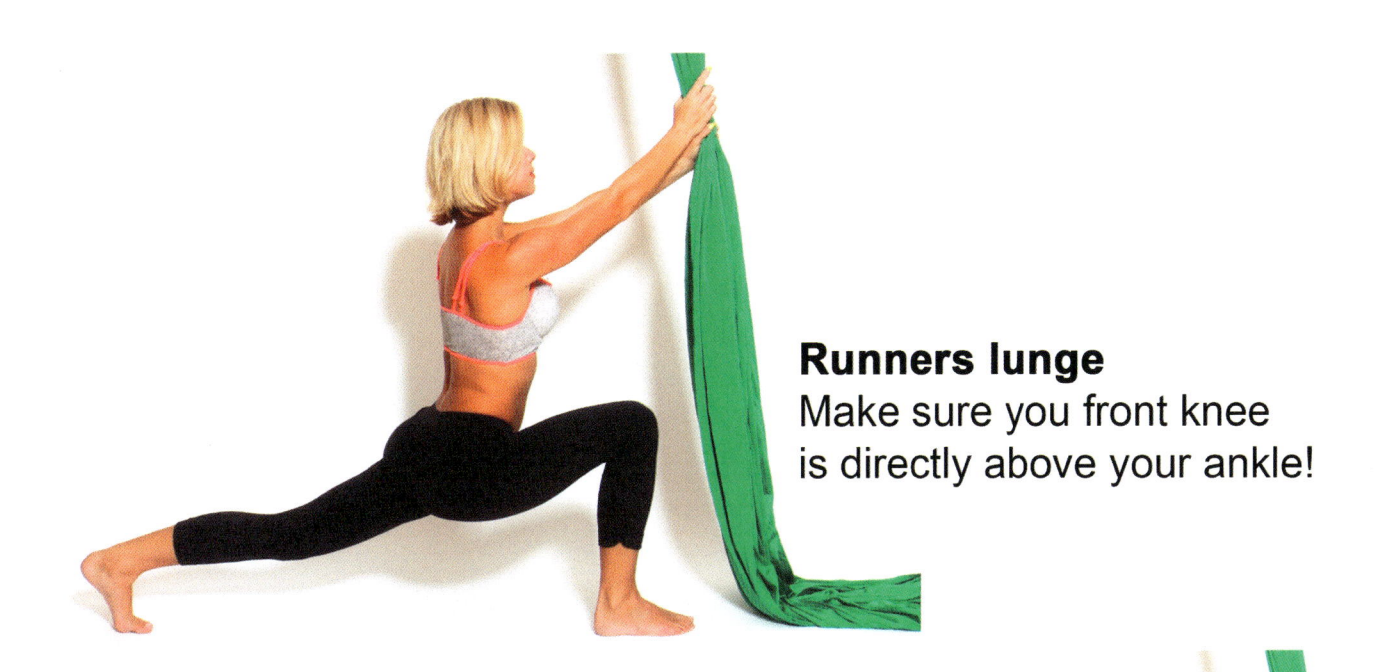

Runners lunge
Make sure you front knee is directly above your ankle!

Hamstring stretch
Keep your front foot flexed and your front leg as straight as possible.
Keep your spine elongated so that you have a flat back
(imagine you're touching your belly to your thigh)

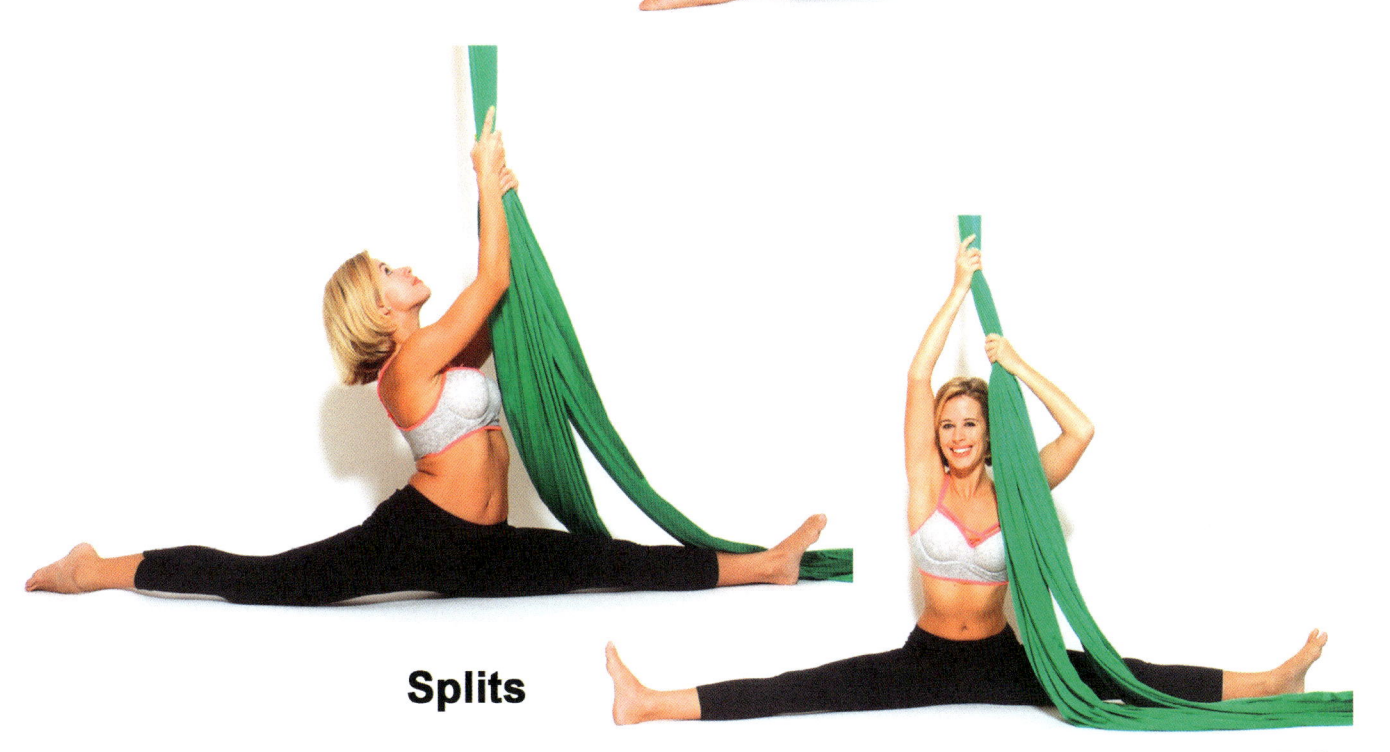

Splits

CHAPTER 2
SINGLE AND DOUBLE FOOTLOCKS

Welcome to the world of footlocks!

A footlock is a wrap that allows you to stand in the fabric without falling out.

When first learning, the fabric will squeeze tightly against the ankle. It can be painful in the beginning so take breaks when needed. The fabric also has a tendancy to tilt the ankle sideways . . . Be aware of this and consciously work on keeping the ankle straight and strong.

DANCER FOOTLOCK
USING YOUR HANDS

ENTRY
Raise your knee and place the fabric against the inside of your thigh. . .

Wrap the fabric under the calf muscle and around the ankle two times.

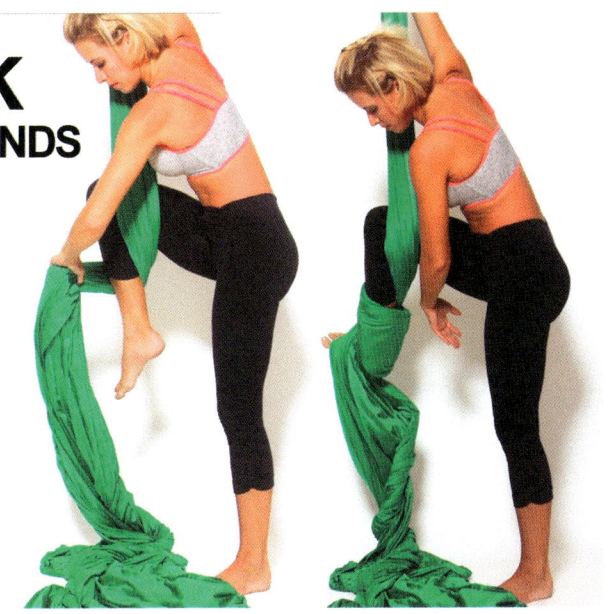

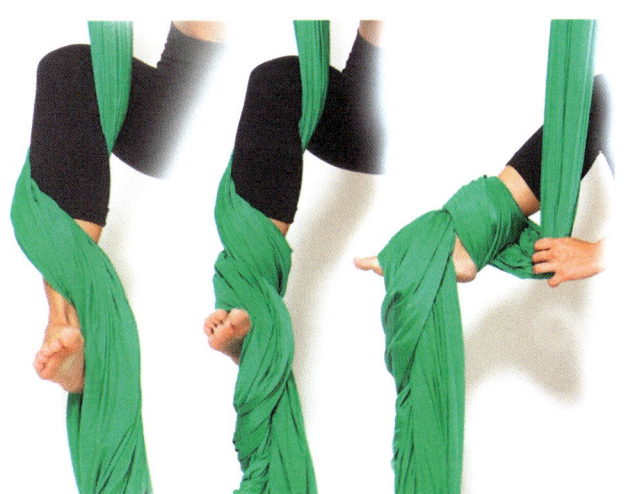

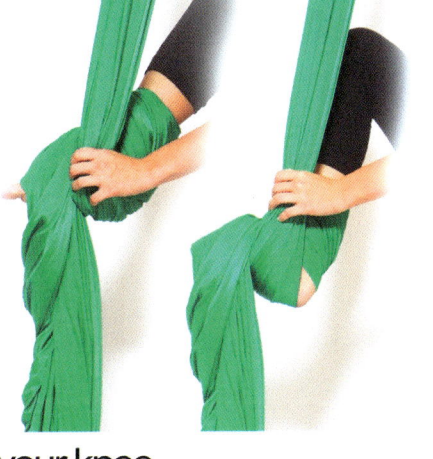

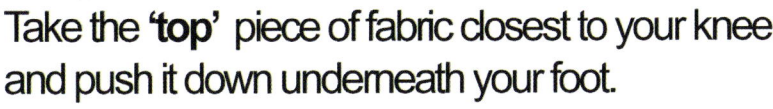

Take the **'top'** piece of fabric closest to your knee and push it down underneath your foot.

Fabric should sit under the sole of your foot . . . slightly closer to the heel.

You may have to lift your foot high into the air to give yourself the slack to get the **'top'** piece under the heel.

EXIT
Point your toes and slide your foot forward off the fabric. (keeping the 'pole' of the fabric in between your thighs)

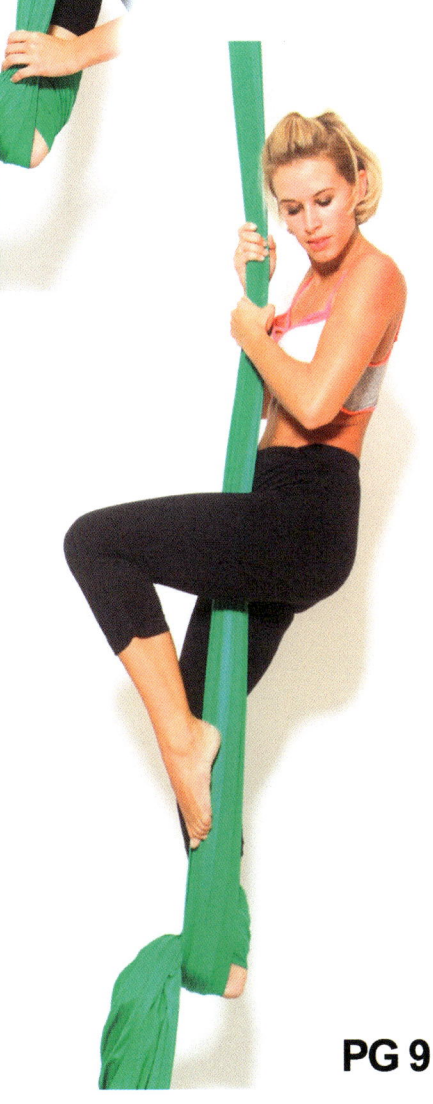

DANCER FOOTLOCK
USING FEET

ENTRY
Once you've wrapped the fabric twice around the ankle . . .
Extend the wrapped foot straight out in front of you . . . .
Grab the fabric high above your head . . .
Lift your free leg off the floor and use it to push the 'pole' of the fabric down the calf and underneath the heel.

EXIT
Bend your knee, point your toes lift your foot up slightly and slide your foot forward off the fabric.

PG 10

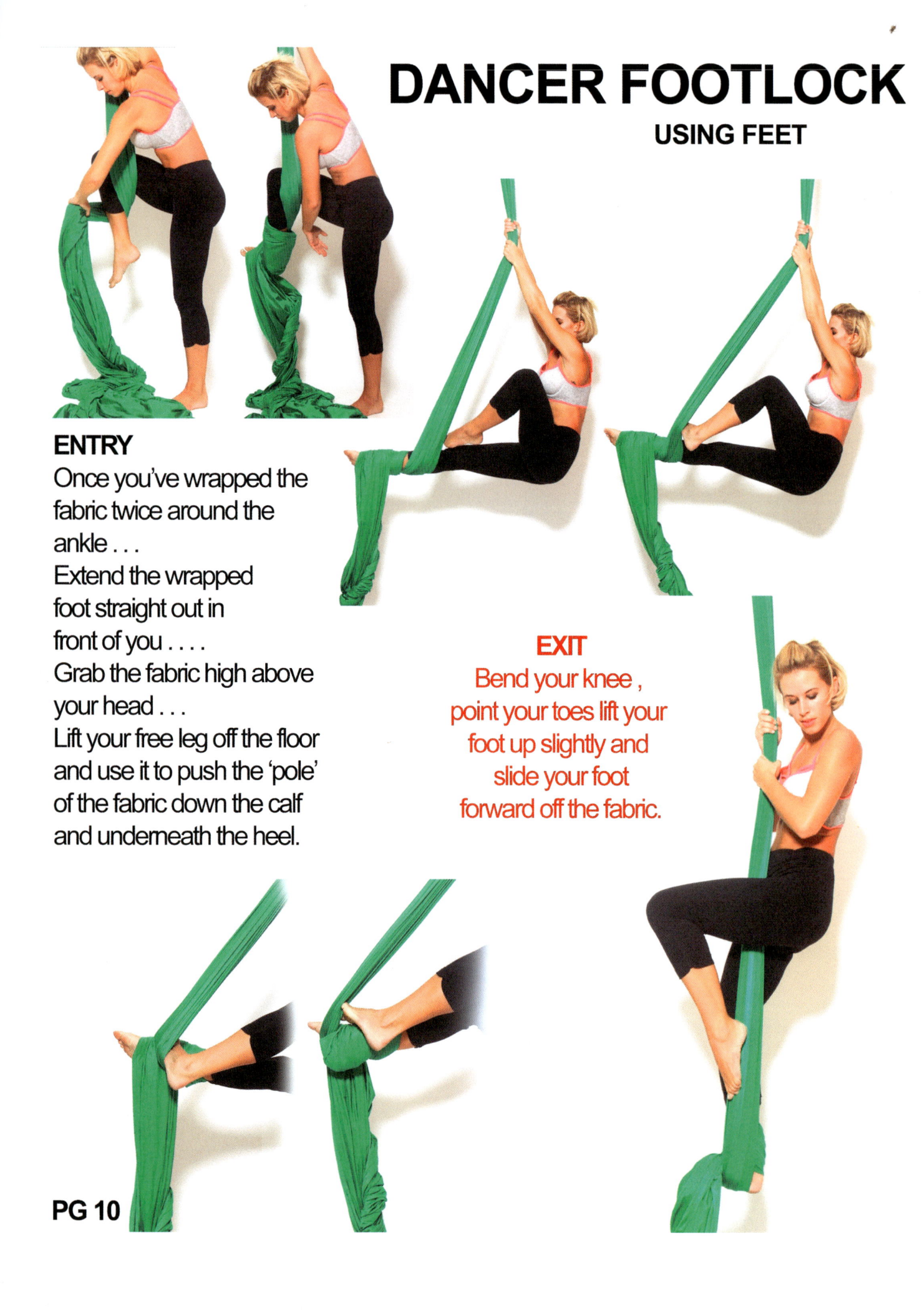

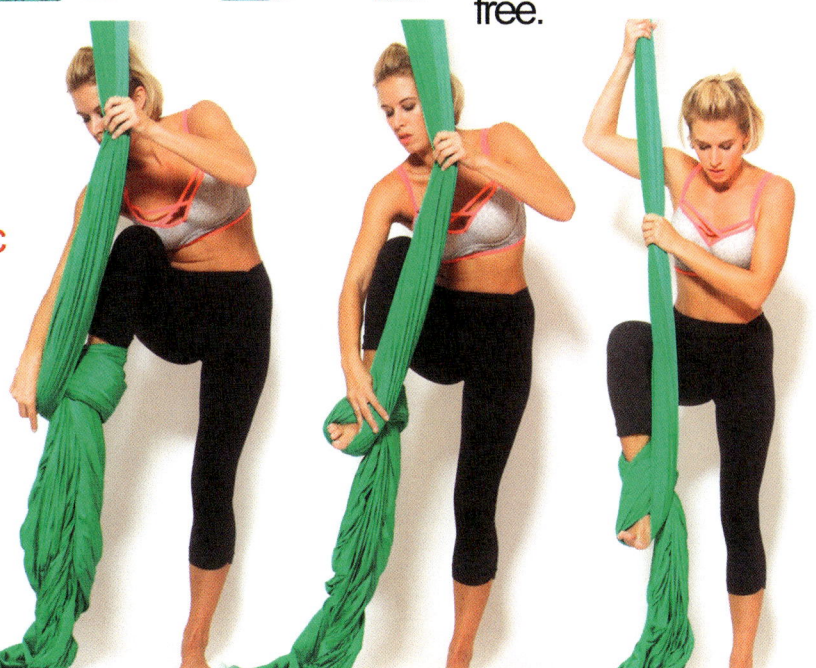

FIGURE 8 FOOTLOCK
USING HANDS

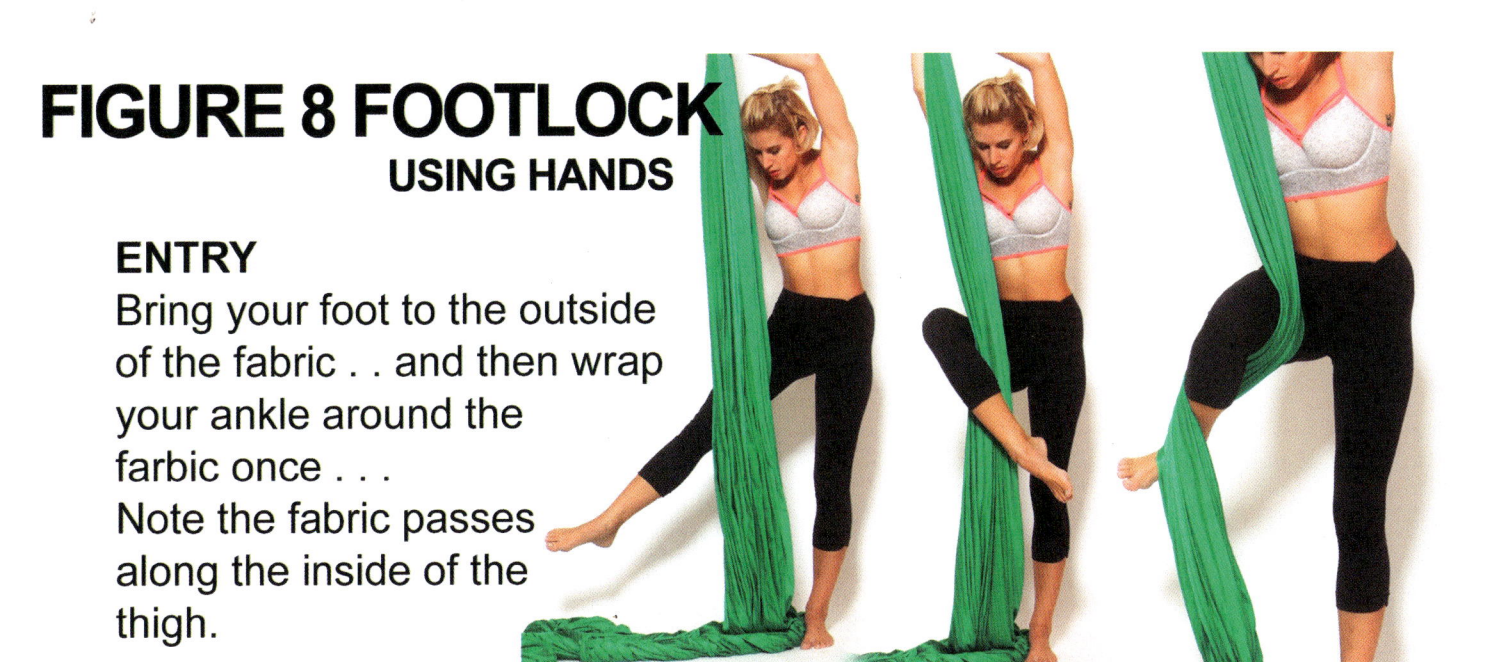

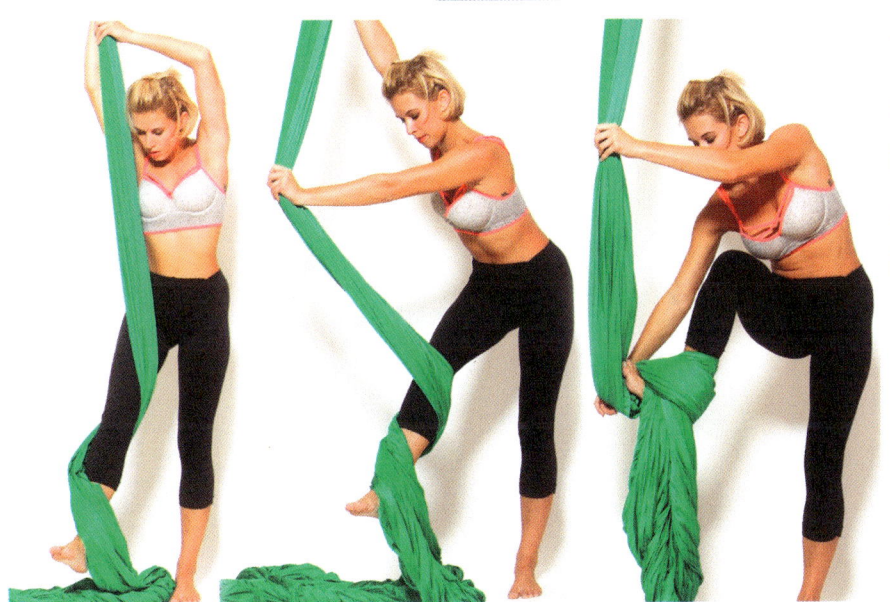

ENTRY
Bring your foot to the outside of the fabric . . and then wrap your ankle around the farbic once . . .
Note the fabric passes along the inside of the thigh.

Take the **'pole'** of the fabric and push it across the top and to the outside edge of your foot.

Then wrap the fabric underneath the toes and foot.

Make sure your toes are free.

EXIT
Lean back, flex your toes and let the fabric slide from under the foot to the tops of your toes and then off completely.

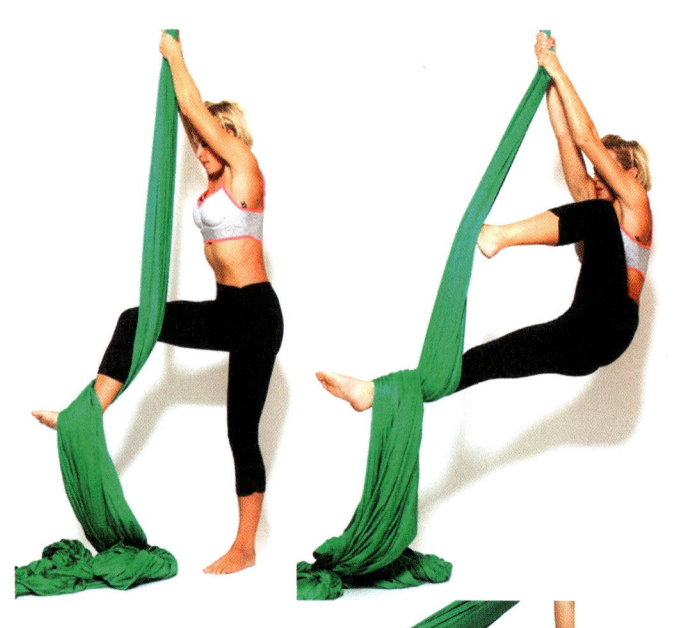

FIGURE 8 FOOTLOCK
NO HANDS

ENTRY
Begin by wrapping your ankle once around the fabric . . . from there hold the fabric high above your head . . . and hold your wrapped leg straight out in front of you.

from there . . . lift your free leg into the air and place it high on the fabric . .
(toes facing in)

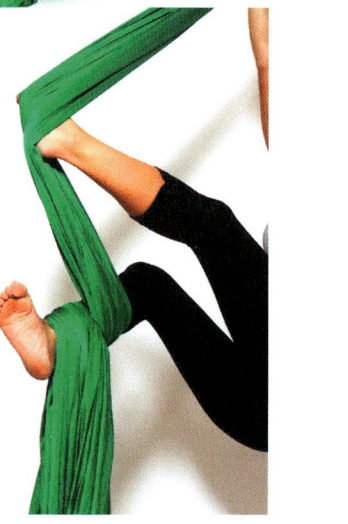

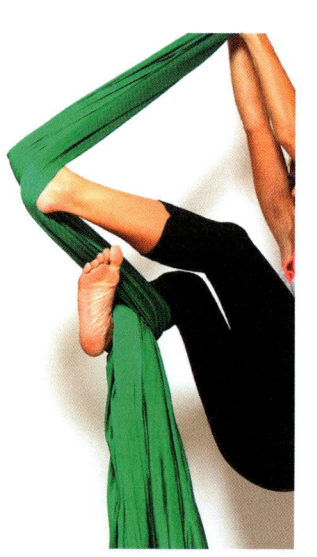

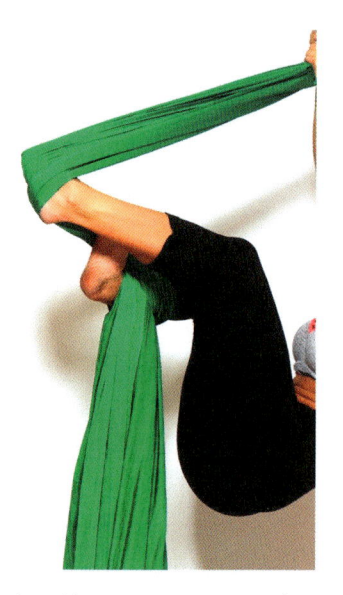

Keeping your foot high on the fabric . . . begin to rotate the wrapped foot in towards the body and around the fabric so that the sole of your foot steps into the fabric.

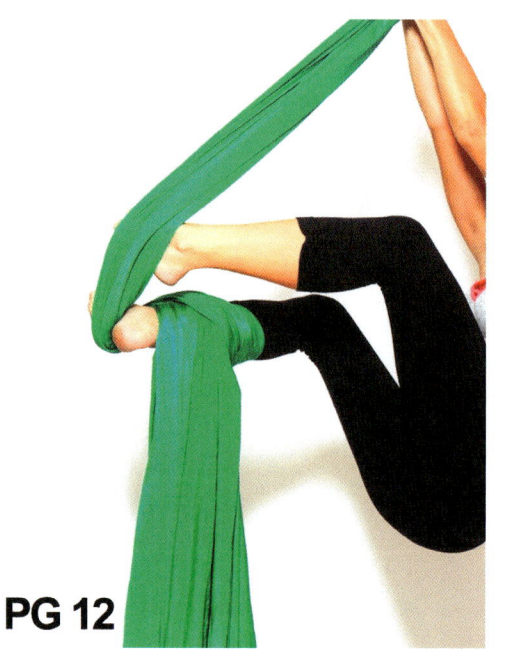

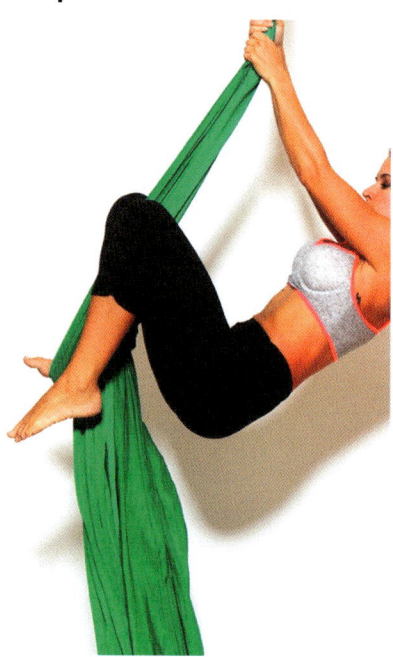

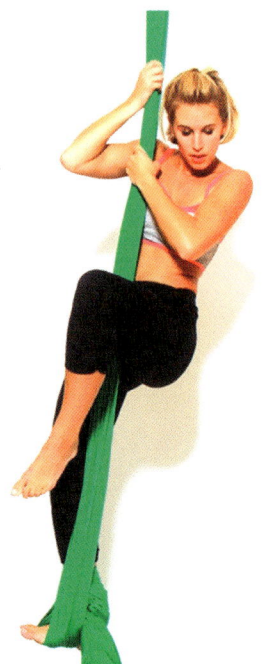

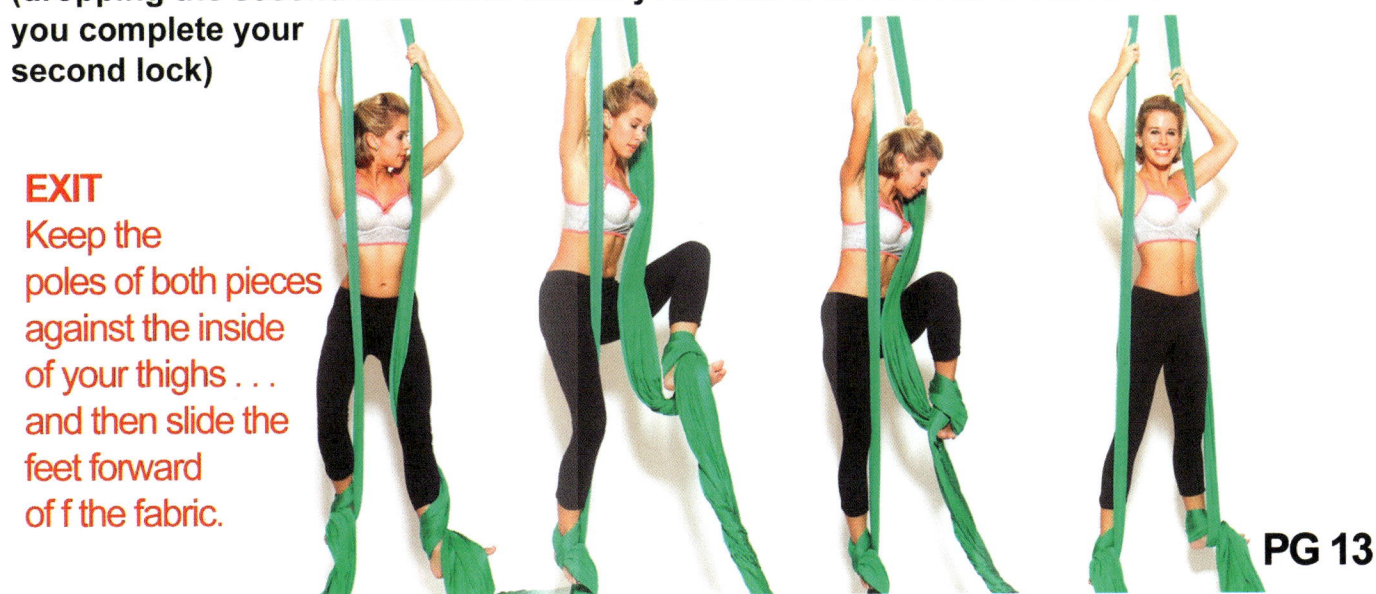

DOUBLE FOOTLOCK
USING HANDS

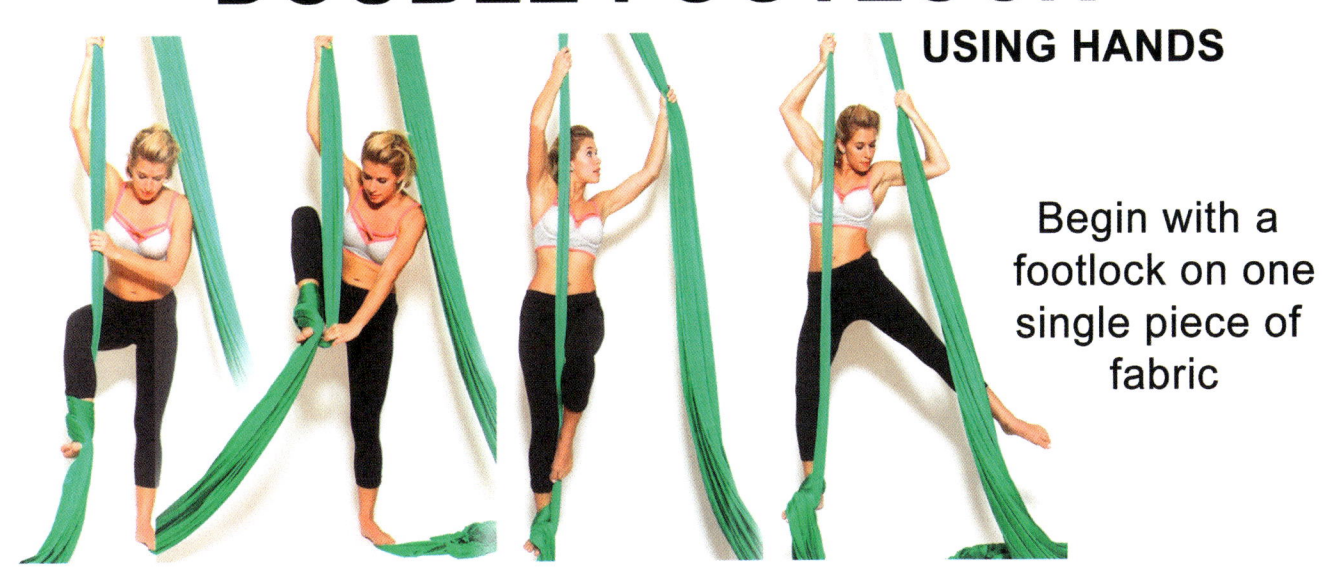

Begin with a footlock on one single piece of fabric

Reach up high, stand on the fabric and bring the free piece to the free side.

Wrap the free fabric twice around your free leg . . . before stepping into the lock, slide your leg down the fabric so it is slightly lower than your first foot.

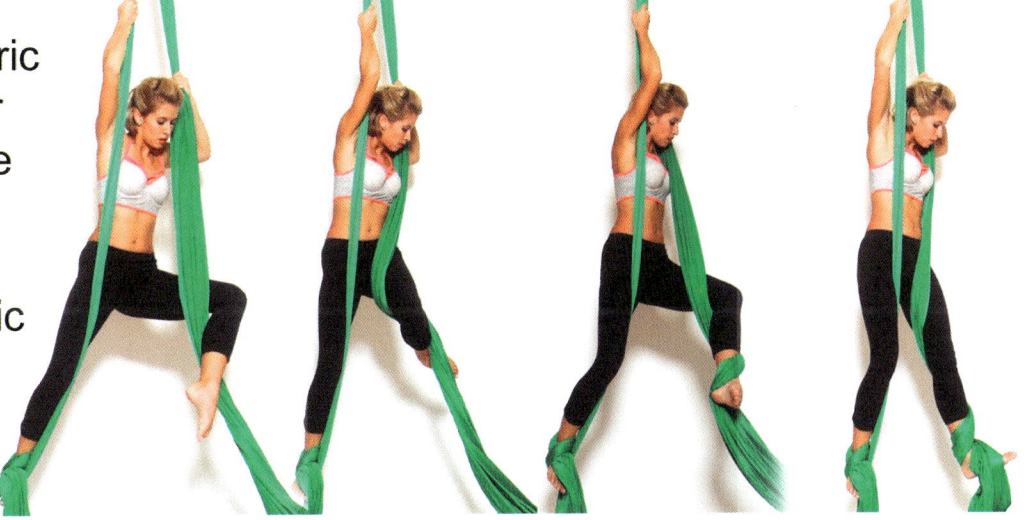

(dropping the second foot lower allows you to have more even footlocks once you complete your second lock)

EXIT
Keep the poles of both pieces against the inside of your thighs . . . and then slide the feet forward of f the fabric.

DOUBLE FOOTLOCKS NO HANDS

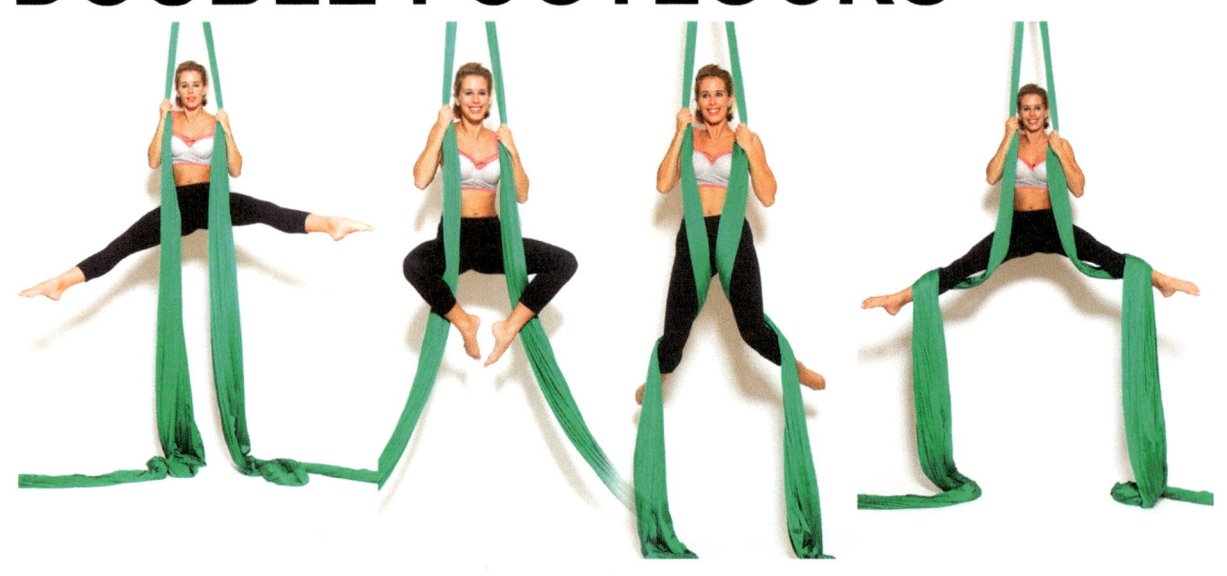

Split the fabric, pull up with your legs in a straddle and then wrap your legs around the fabric **two times**.

As soon as you have the double wrap squeeze your legs together.

(this will help you from losing grip and sliding down the fabric)

Reach up, pull your knees up and step your feet into the slack created.

EXIT
Keep the fabric on the inside of your thighs and slide your feet forward and off the fabric.

CHAPTER 3
WRIST WRAP POSES

"There is a vitality, a life force, an energy, a quickening, that is translated through you into action, and because there is only one of you in all time, this expression is unique."
Martha Graham

Wrist wraps are a great way to build wrist tolerance, arm strength, inversion awareness, balance and tighten your core. Here are few things to know before practicing . . .

1. They can hurt - Remember your body may not be used to the fabric so the pressure around the wrists can be intense. Try to remember to use more grip with the hands and to rest less weight on the wrists in the fabric.

2. Wrapping the fabric twice is the most common method, but you have the option of wrapping more or not wrapping at all if you wish to develop more grip strength.

3. You can lose grip strength faster than you think so come down if you feel out of strength and be sure to practice your first few with padding underneath.

4. It is easy to go too far and backflip all the way through the fabric. backflipping through can be very dangerous as it puts the shoulders in a very precarious position.

DANCER WRIST WRAP

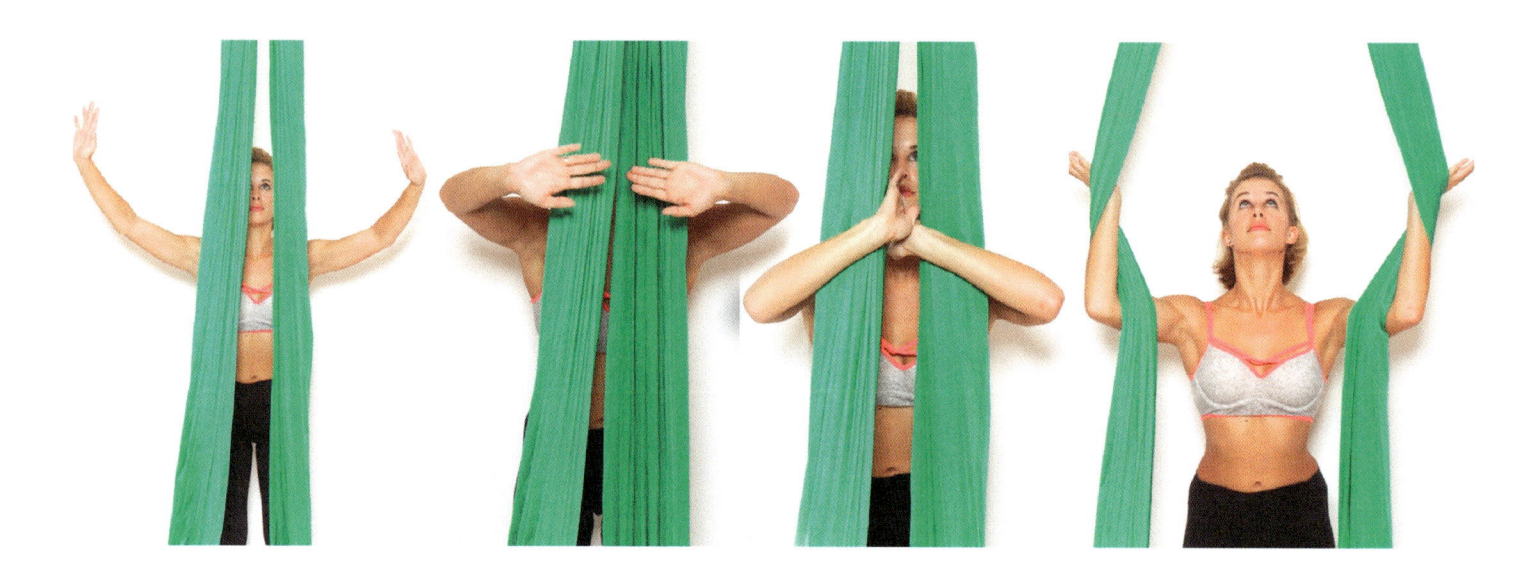

ENTRY
Stand behind the fabric, wrap your hands wide around the outside and then to the front. From there bring them in towards your body. . .
DO THIS TWICE.

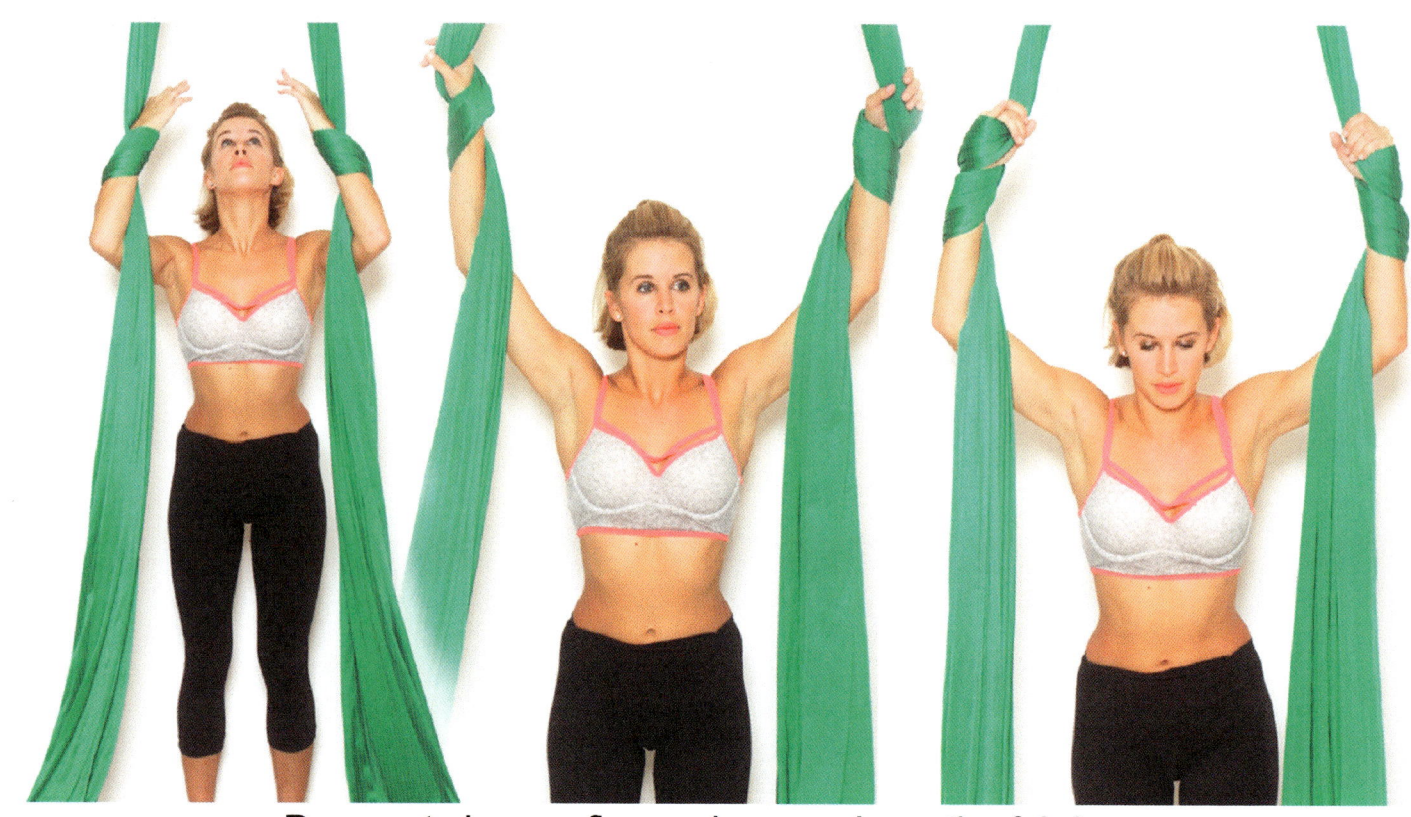

Be sure to have a firm and even grip on the fabric.

BASIC POSES FROM A WRIST WRAP

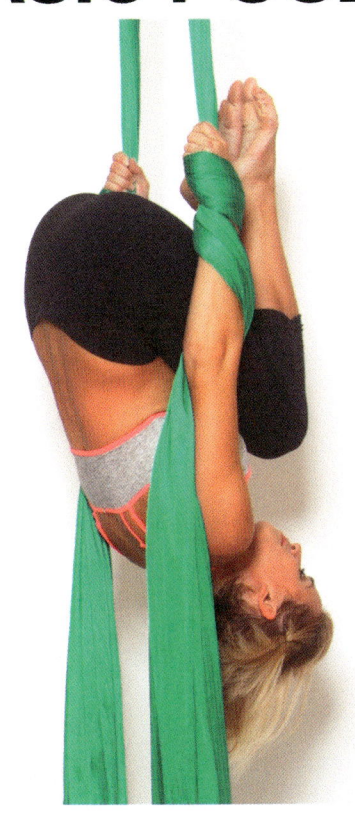

TUCK
Pull your knees to your chest . . . drop your chest back and straighten your arms.

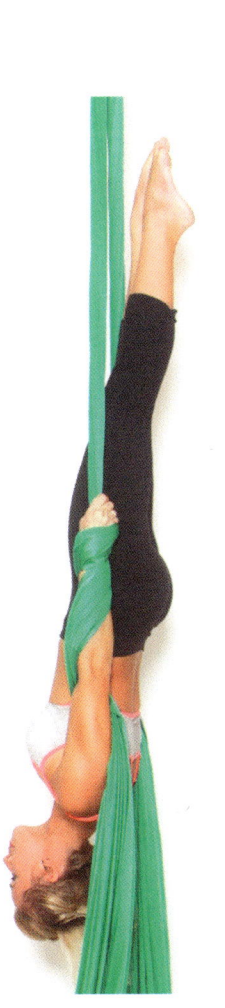

PIKE
From a tuck position straighten out your legs.

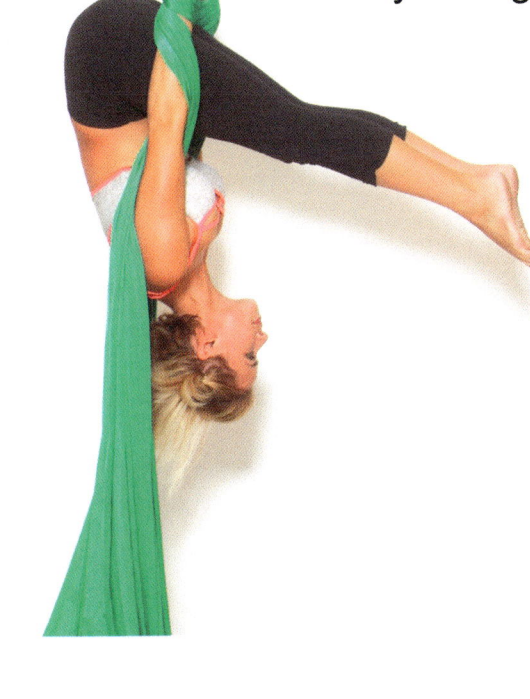

PENCIL
From a pike raise your legs straight up towards the ceiling.

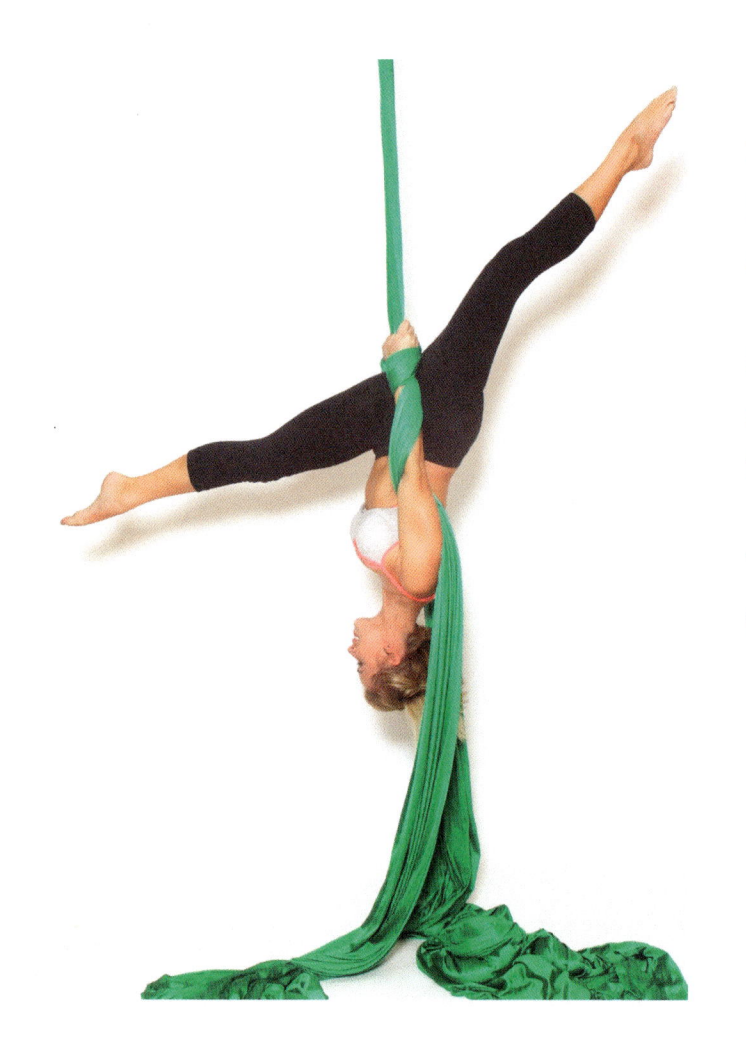

SPLIT

From a pencil . . open your legs into a split.

If you have balance issues here . . . arch your back and look to the floor.

Try to keep your hips in between the fabric.

STAG

From a split . . . bend each knee about 90 degrees.

WORD OF CAUTION

Always be sure to come out of this the same way you came in....

Think booty to the floor . . . some people have a tendancy to want to flip all the way through the fabric and this can dislocate or put the shoulders in a very akward position.

BIRDS NEST

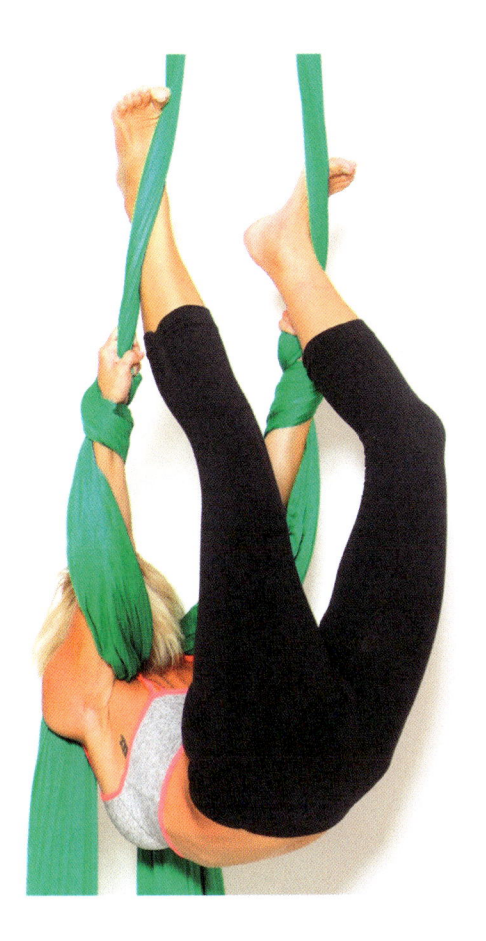

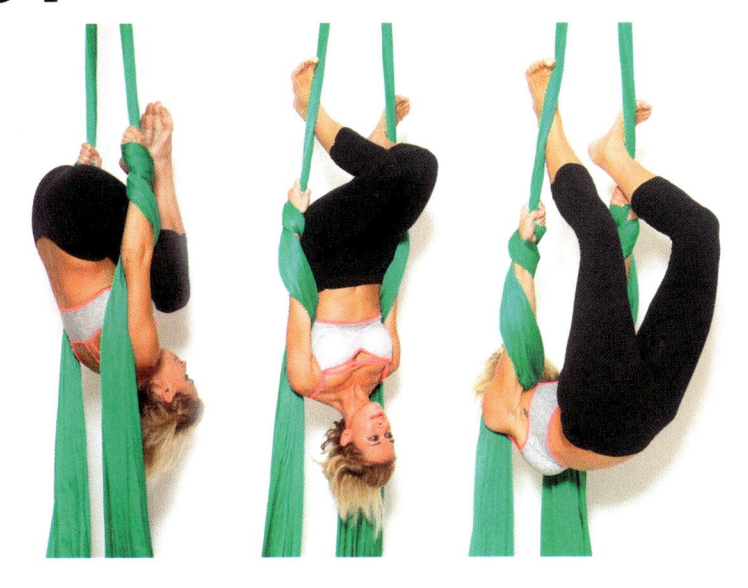

ENTRY
From a tuck . . . hook the tops of your toes against the back of the fabric. (note how the knees are still together and in between the fabric)

From here drive your hips forward and arch your back.

SAFETY CONCERNS
Be mindful of your toes so they don't slip off the fabric. . . keeping them flexed will help with this.

Remember to come back the way you came in . . . back to a tuck then booty to the floor.

SPLIT THROUGH

ENTRY
From a birds nest . . . allow one leg to unwrap and extend down to the floor.

You can keep the leg bent or straight.

Tips / Techniques
Remember to place your free leg back against the fabric to come out.

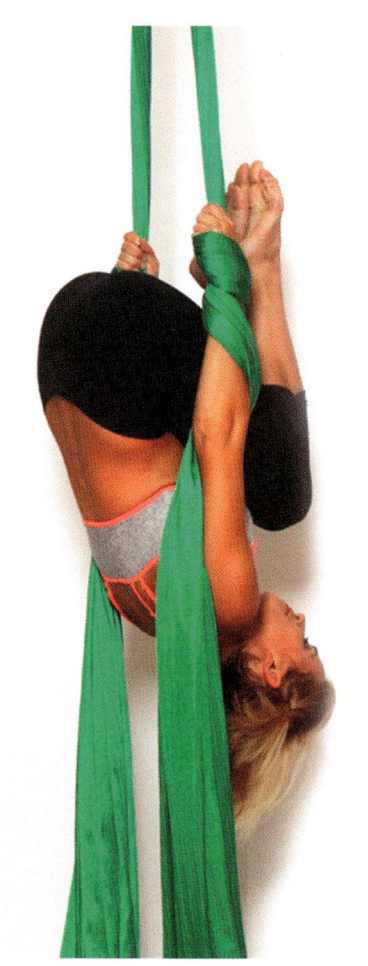

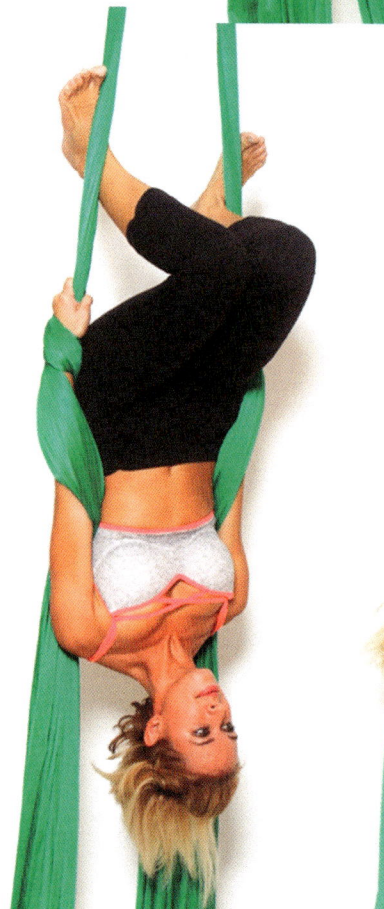

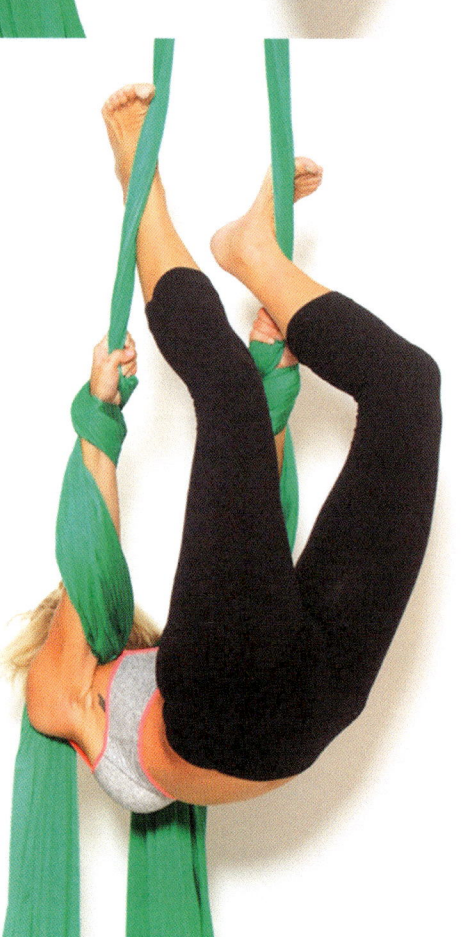

PIGEON FROM WRIST WRAP

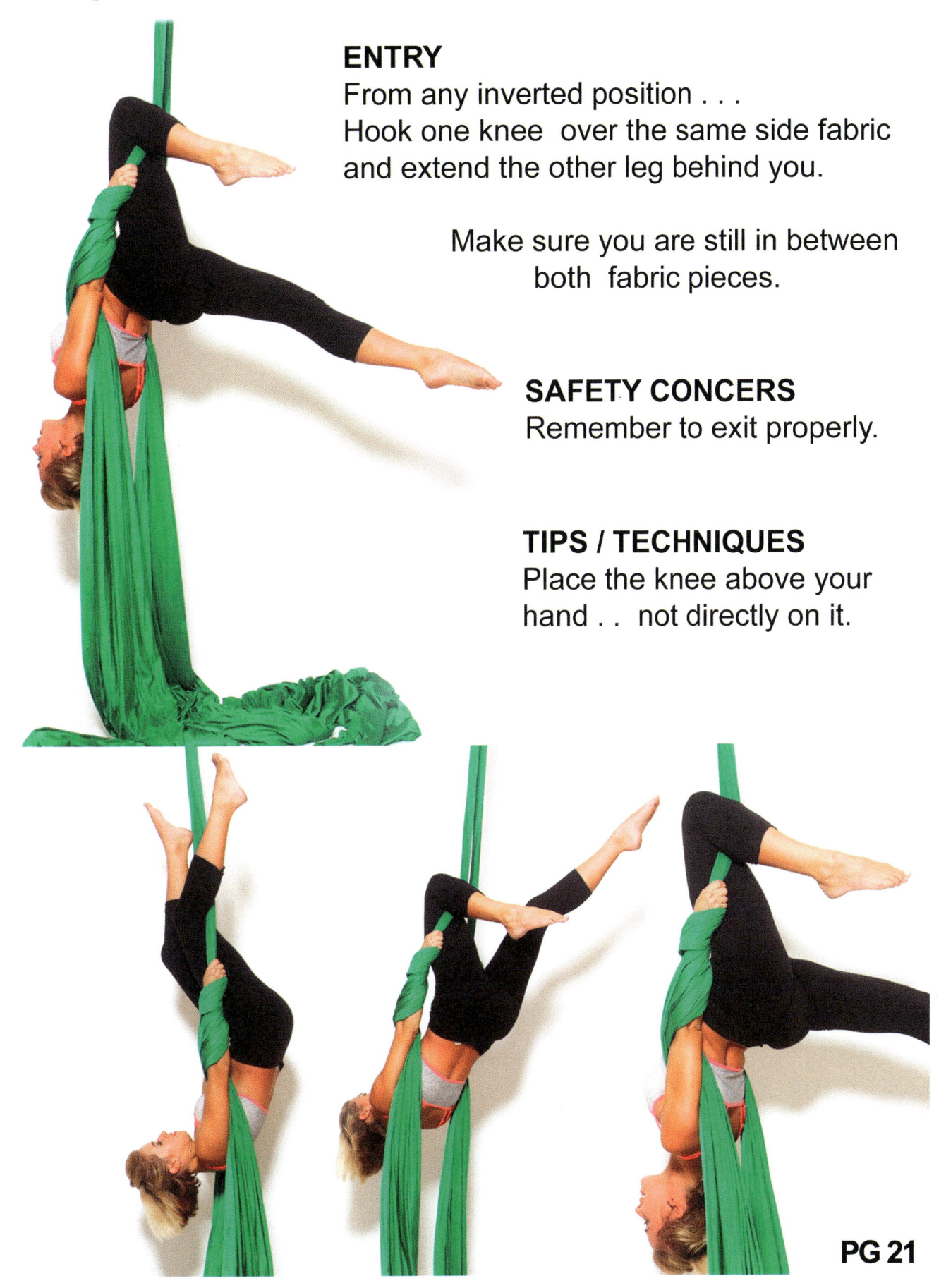

ENTRY
From any inverted position . . .
Hook one knee over the same side fabric and extend the other leg behind you.

Make sure you are still in between both fabric pieces.

SAFETY CONCERS
Remember to exit properly.

TIPS / TECHNIQUES
Place the knee above your hand . . not directly on it.

PG 21

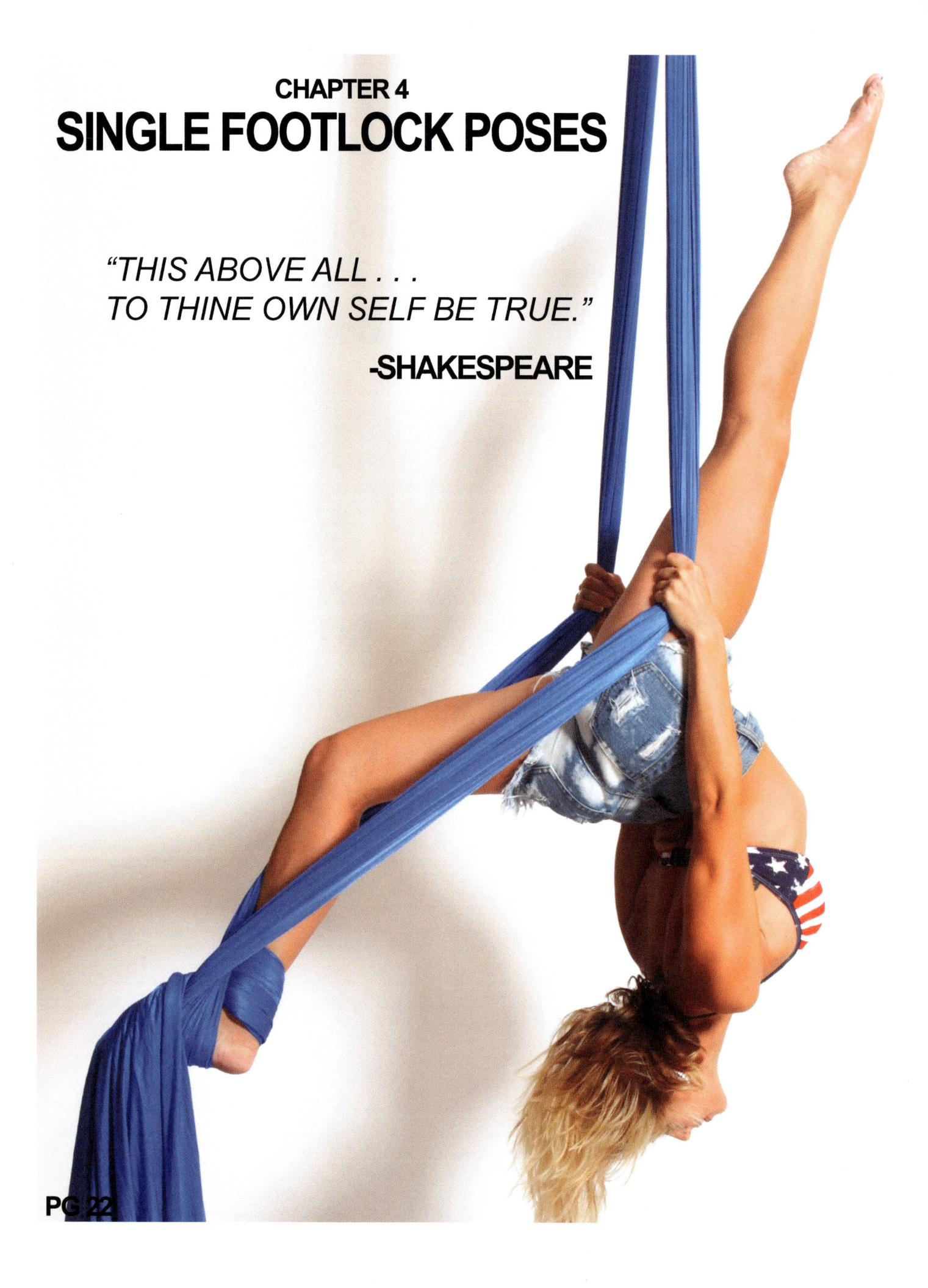

CHAPTER 4
SINGLE FOOTLOCK POSES

*"THIS ABOVE ALL . . .
TO THINE OWN SELF BE TRUE."*
             -SHAKESPEARE

LADY SIT

ENTRY
From a single footlock, begin to squat down and cross the free leg over your "locked" leg. Keep the fabric in between the thighs and close to the hips.

SAFETY CONCERNS
'Weak footlock' - it is very easy to let the fabric twist your locked ankle off to one side. Keep your locked ankle flexed and strong.

TECHNIQUE / TIPS
Keep the Hips in close to fabric and keep the legs crossed tight .. LIKE A LADY!

VARIATIONS

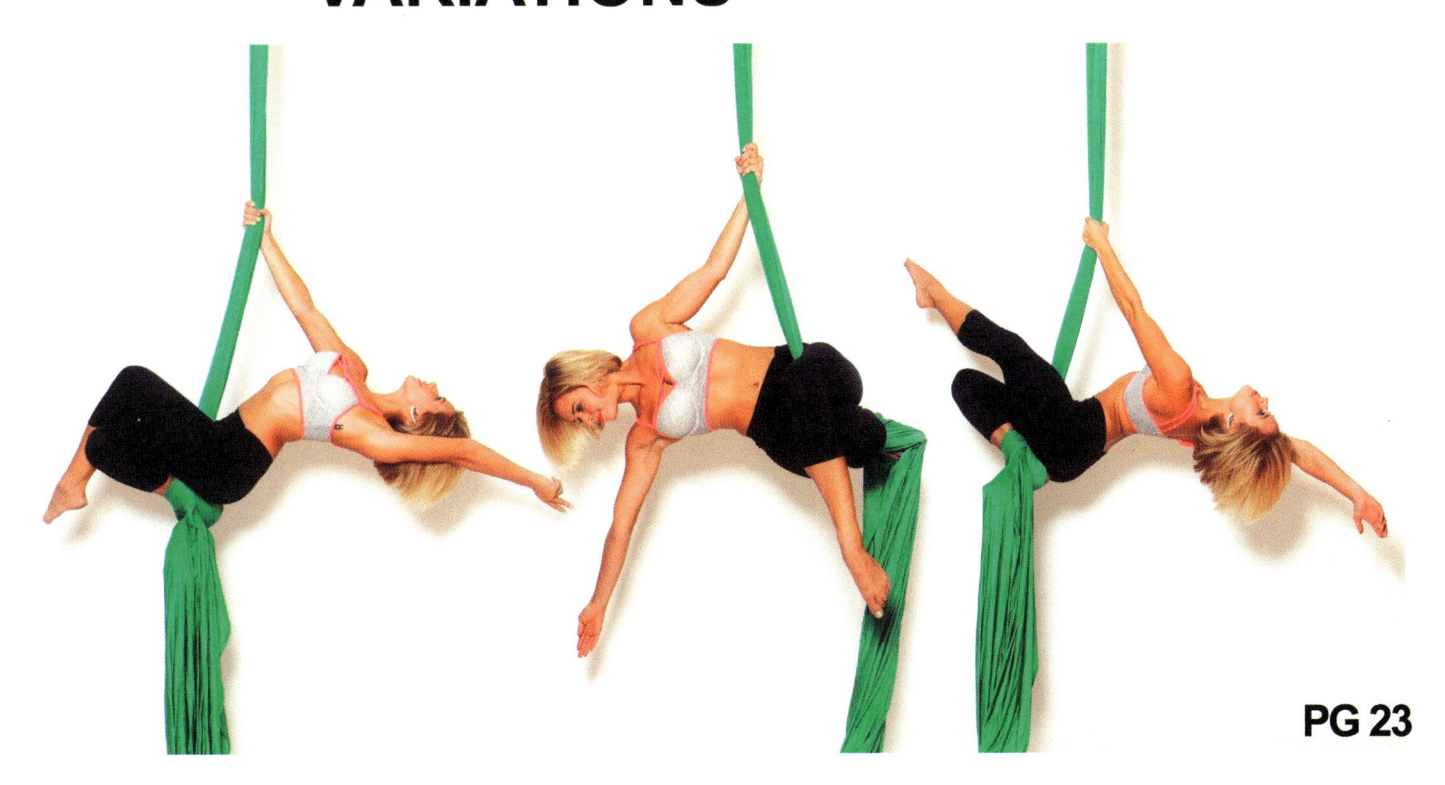

PG 23

DRAMA QUEEN

ENTRY
From a single footlock , bend and raise your free leg. Keep your hips close to the fabric and arch your back.

SAFTEY CONCERNS
Be mindful of your grip on the fabric so as not to slip.

TECHNIQUES / TIPS
Keep your hips close to the fabric.

ATTITUDE

ENTRY
From a single footlock, raise your free leg. Keep your hips close to the fabric and arch your back.

SAFTEY CONCERNS
Be mindful of your grip on the fabric so as not to slip.

TECHNIQUES / TIPS
Keep your hips close to fabric.

NOTE: YOU COULD ALWAYS DO THIS POSE WITH YOUR ELBOW HOOKED AROUND THE FABRIC IF YOUR HAND GRIP IS WEAK.

TURNOUT

ENTRY
From a single footlock, reach both hands high above your head. Extend your free leg out to the side. . . then turn your body 180 degrees in that direction.

(IF YOUR FREE LEG IS YOUR LEFT LEG THEN TURN LEFT . . . IF RIGHT, THEN TURN RIGHT)

SAFETY CONCERNS
Be aware of your grip strength!

TECHNIQUES / TIPS
You can turn in either direction, but it is simpler to turn towards the free leg.

Hands can reposition / regrip once the body is turned out, or they can stay in your original start position.

(WHICH CAN TWIST THE ARMS IN AN UNCOMFORTABLE POSITION IF YOU ARE NOT VERY SHOULDER FLEXIBLE.)

Head sits in between arms while you are turning out and once you have turned out.

Always hold the fabric high above your head.

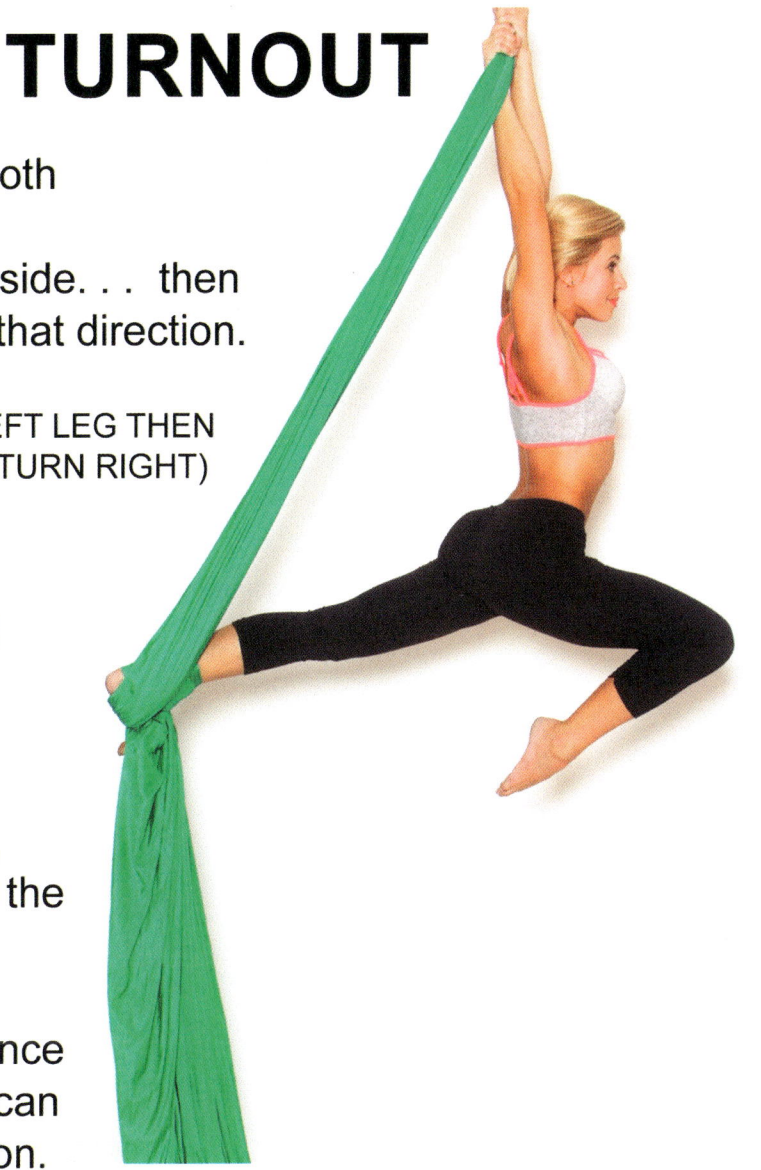

STAR TURNOUT

ENTRY
From a single footlock, reach your same side arm high on the fabric.

(IF YOUR RIGHT FOOT IS LOCKED THEN YOUR RIGHT HAND IS THE SAME SIDE HAND)

Point your free leg out to the side and then slowly lower your body out and towards your free leg.

SAFETY CONCERNS
It is very easy to overestimate your grip strength so lower slowly into your turnout.

TECHNIQUES / TIPS
Hold high on the fabric.

Turnout slowly so as not to peel off the fabric.

You can also use your elbow to hold the fabric if your grip is not solid.

As a variation you can grab your free leg with your free hand and extend into a split stretch.

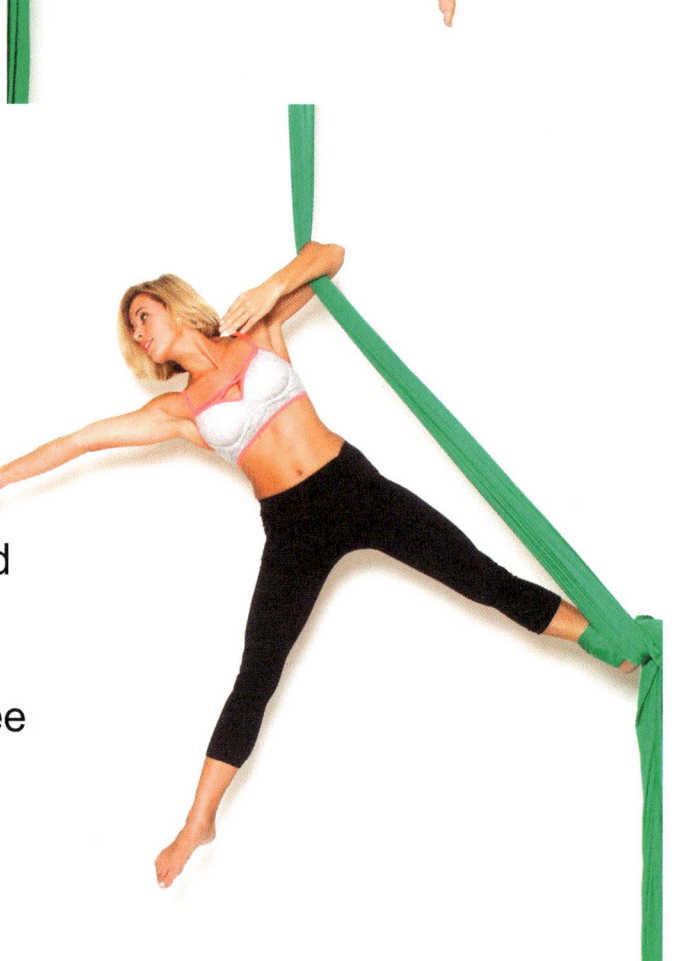

SHOULDER DROP THROUGHS

ENTRY: 'REVERSE'
From a single footlock, split the fabric into two pieces and stand with your hips / body in between them . . .
Bring only your shoulders and armpits to the front side of the fabric so that the fabric rests against the back of your shoulders, then allow your body to drop backwards. Your shoulders will slide down the fabric slightly so be aware of rope burn.

NOTE
The difference in where the fabric sits in the arms for each pose.
reverse = fabric behind shoulders
forward = fabric in armpits

TECHNIQUES / TIPS
Sleeves work best with this pose as fabric can burn the skin.

The lower you sink down, the harder it is to get back up.

ENTRY: 'FORWARD'
From a single footlock, split the fabric and stand in between the two pieces.
Keep the fabric resting against the front of your armpits and allow only your body / hips to drop forward through the fabric.

'REVERSE'

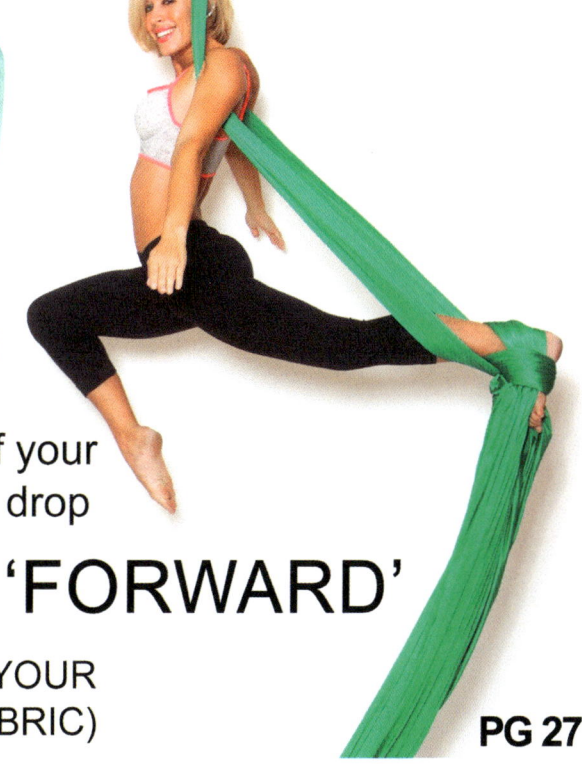

'FORWARD'

(AGAIN BE AWARE OF ROPE BURN AS YOUR ARMPITS SLIDE LOWER DOWN THE FABRIC)

FORWARD PENDULUM

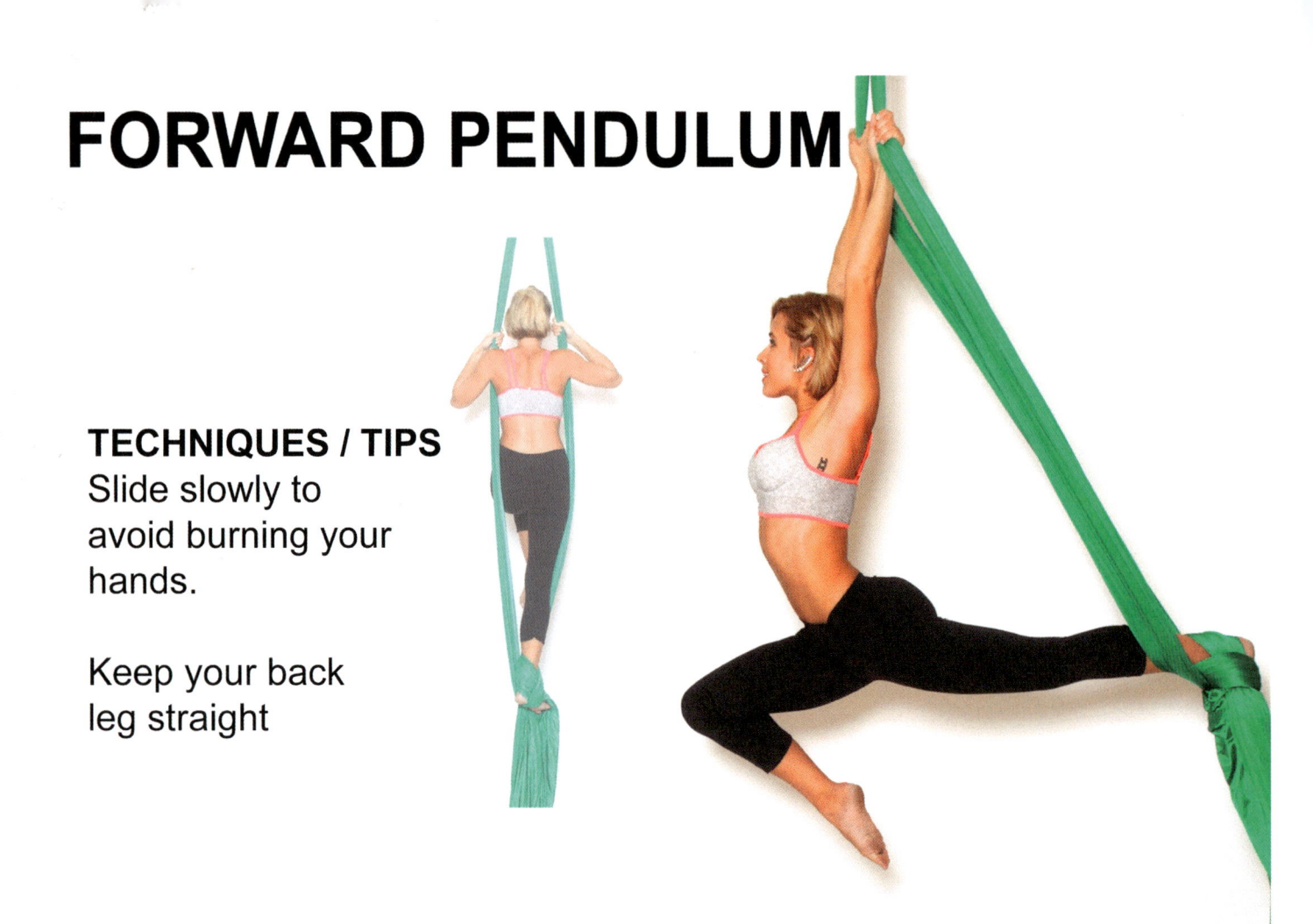

TECHNIQUES / TIPS
Slide slowly to avoid burning your hands.

Keep your back leg straight

ENTRY
From a single footlock, split the fabric and set your hips in between the two pieces . . . Slide your hands up the fabric (without changing grip) and hold high above your head (thumbs will be facing up).

Allow your whole body (including your arms) to slide through the fabric and lower down until the back is arched (in most cases your palms / wrists will turn out slightly).

To exit just pull your body back up with your arms!

SAFETY CONCERNS
Not being strong enough to pull yourself back up.

Lower yourself down halfway to test your arm strength.

PG 28

REVERSE PENDULUM

ENTRY
From a single footlock, split the fabric and bring your hips in between the two pieces.

Slide your hands down so you're holding the fabric at your hip level. (thumbs up)

Keep your supporting leg straight and begin to lean back. as you lean back, straighten out your arms, look back for the floor and drive your hips up to the ceiling.

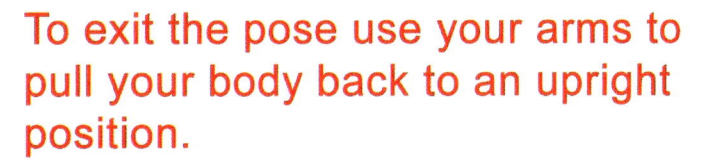

To exit the pose use your arms to pull your body back to an upright position.

SAFETY CONCERNS
It is possible to go too far backwards and flip over. . . This usually happens when you flip back too fast or if your hands are super low on the fabric.

TECHNIQUES / TIPS
Straighten your arms when in the pose to take save your muscle strength.

The lower your initial grip on the fabric the furthur upside down you will go.

As a variation you can straighten your free leg into a split, however this changes your center of gravity so do it slowly to avoid flipping over.

DANCER

ENTRY
From a single footlock
adjust your hand positioning first ...
Your same side hand goes in between your
chest and the fabric and regrips the fabric above your
head in an upward facing grip (palm up) ...

Then bring your whole body to the 'front' side
of the fabric (so the fabric is resting at your back).

Re-adjust your grip so that the fabric is inside your
opposite side armpit.
Extend your free leg and drive your hips out to the
side to keep the fabric across your lower back.
Your free hand then grabs your free ankle and
extends into dancers pose.

SAFETY CONCERNS
Balance - if the fabric is not tucked between your
armpit you will have no balance and fall forward.

EXIT
Regrip the fabric
and unwind your body
back the way it came.

TECHNIQUES / TIPS
The fabric must be against your lower back. not your booty.
When twisting around the fabric keep your hands high above your head level.

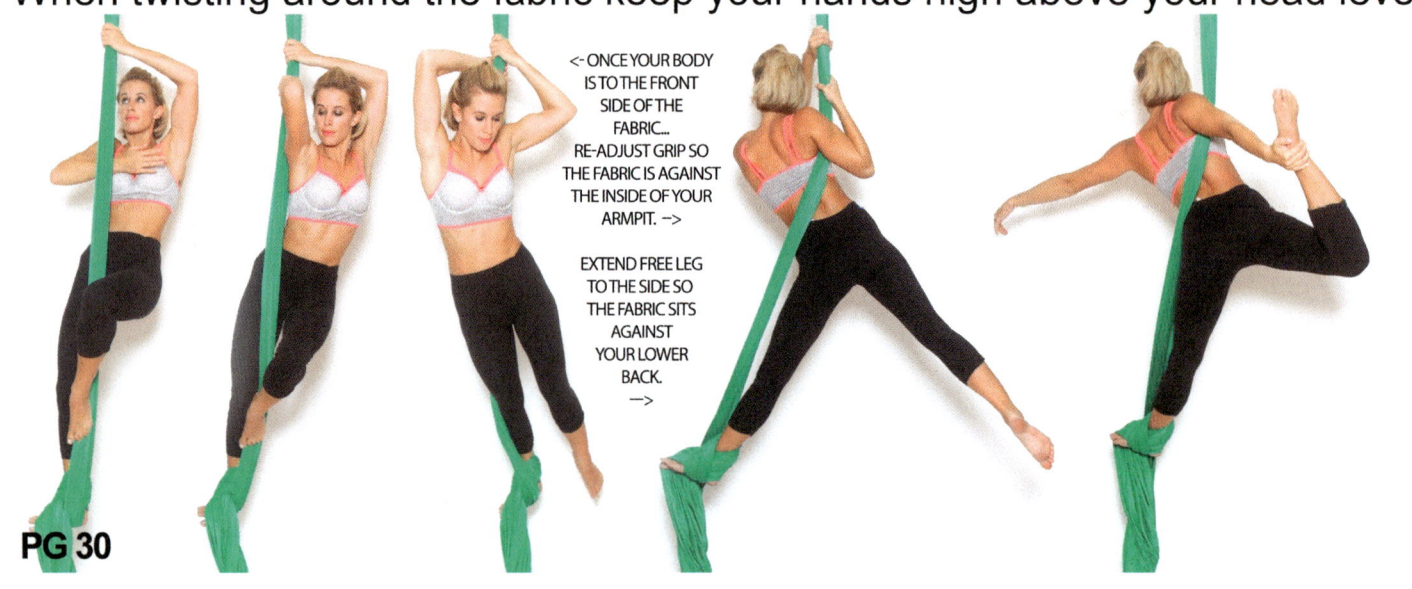

<- ONCE YOUR BODY IS TO THE FRONT SIDE OF THE FABRIC... RE-ADJUST GRIP SO THE FABRIC IS AGAINST THE INSIDE OF YOUR ARMPIT. ->

EXTEND FREE LEG TO THE SIDE SO THE FABRIC SITS AGAINST YOUR LOWER BACK. -->

BOW AND ARROW

ENTRY
From a single footlock, split the fabric into two pieces and bring your hips in between them ... Keep your armpits against the 'back' side of the fabric and let your free leg / hips go through to the 'front' side of the fabric. extend your leg / hips out to the side and grab your free ankle with your free hand ... push the opposing piece of fabric away from the body.

Note how her hips are all the way to the front & side of the fabric. . .
if the fabric is catching against the booty you will have a hard time completing the pose.

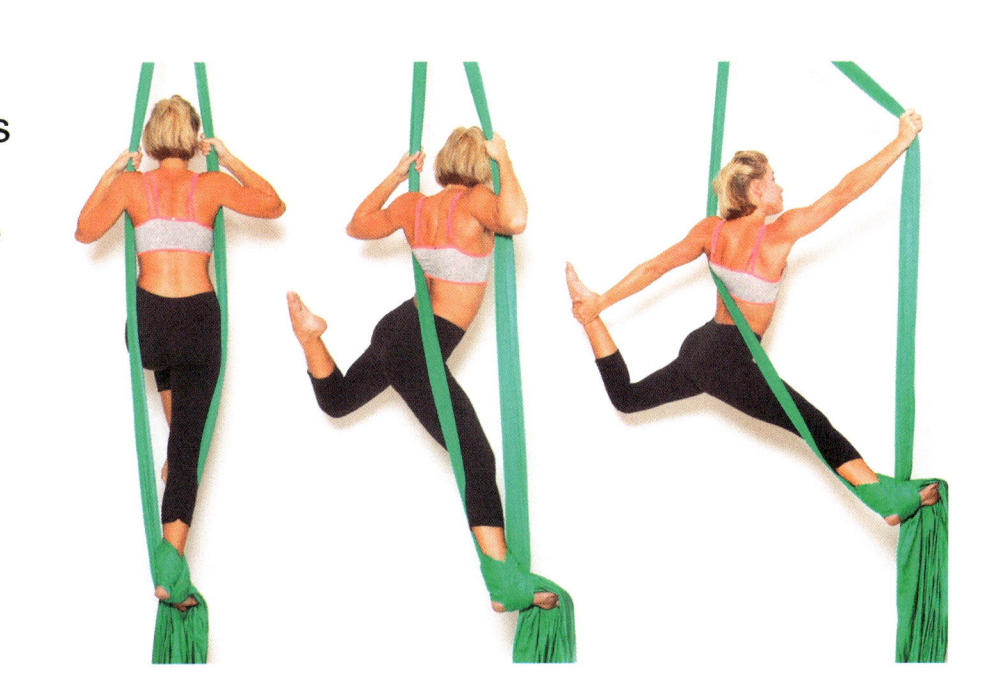

TO EXIT - grab the fabric and pulll your body back in between the two pieces.

SAFETY CONCERNS
Balance - shoulders must be behind the fabric while booty is in front.

TECHNIQUES / TIPS
For best balance you want the fabric across the lower back , sometimes the fabric catches against the booty which inhibits you from 'pushing' the opposing fabric away from the body.

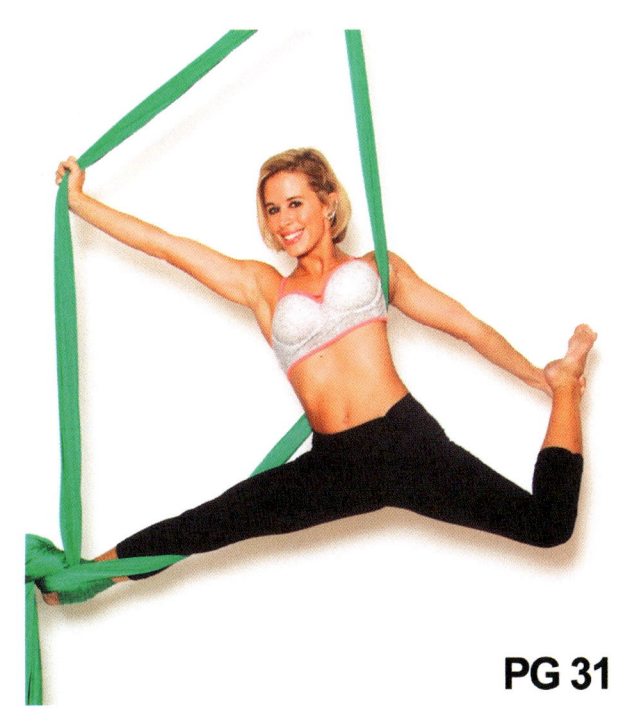

PG 31

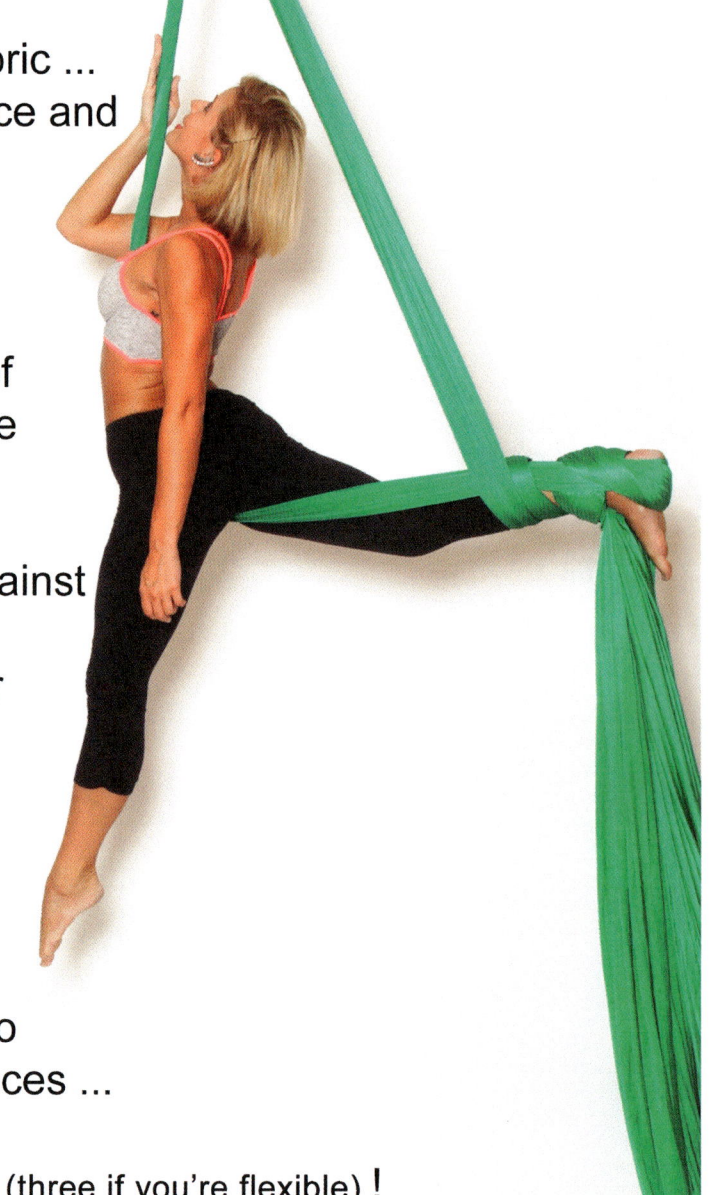

MERMAID

ENTRY

From a single footlock, split the fabric and turn your body sideways in the fabric ... meaning your chest is against one piece and the other piece is at your back ..

(if right foot is locked turn right , if left then turn left)

Lean out of the fabric in the direction of your free leg then turn back to face the fabric.

Take your free leg and place it high against the 'far' piece of fabric (be sure you go over the closer piece and not under it) . (see pic on the opposite page)

Push the far piece down to your ankle (be sure to not push the fabric too far ' as the fabric will slip off the ankle)

and then pull your chest and belly up to rest back in between the two fabric pieces ...

Repeat this process at least two times (three if you're flexible) !

SAFETY CONCERNS

If you don't push the far piece down to the ankle the fabric will squeeze the knee and be very painful.

TECHNIQUES / TIPS

Hold hands high to make it easier to pull yourself into the fabric.

Keep supporting leg as straight and as strong as possible.

PG 32

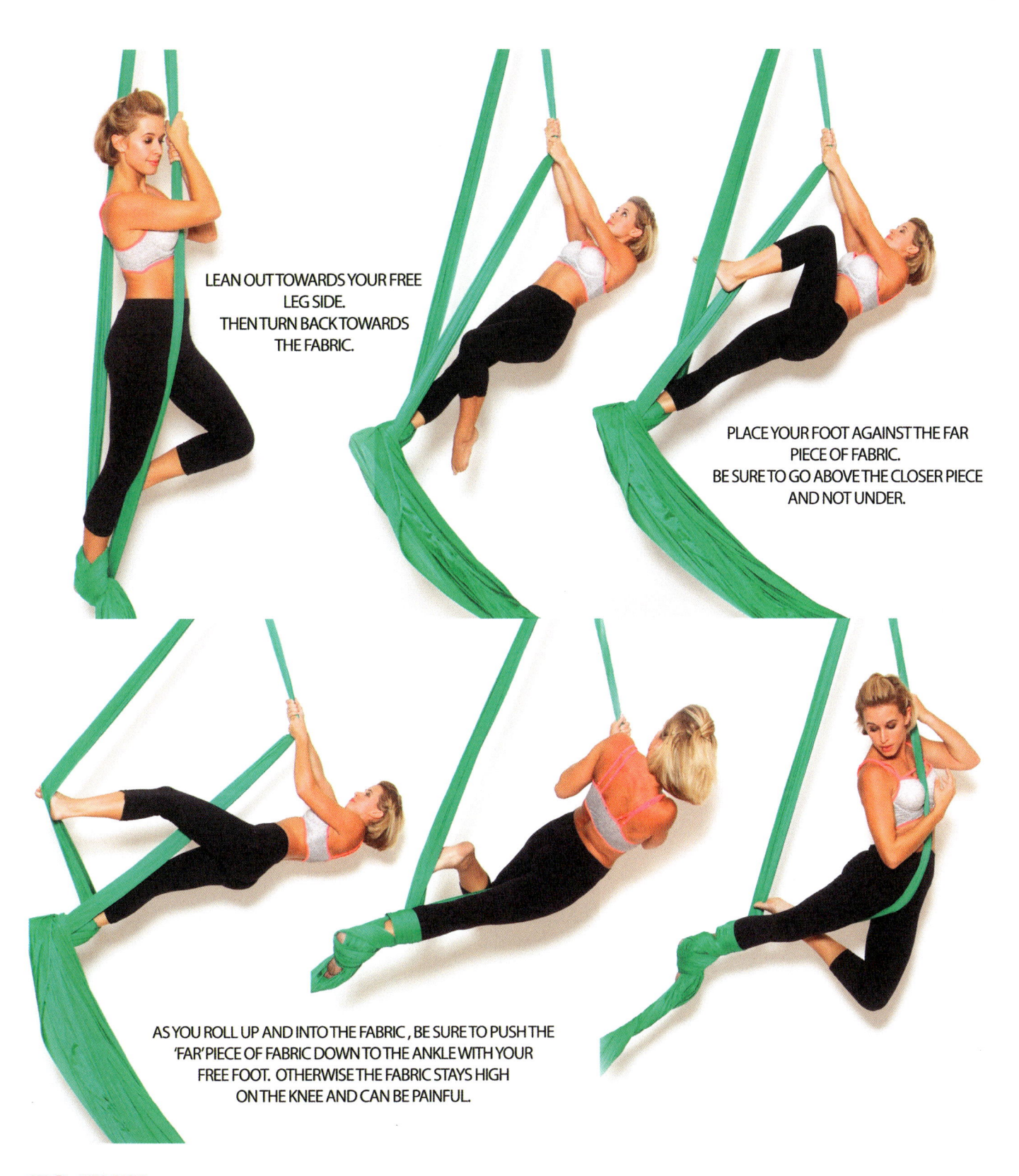

LEAN OUT TOWARDS YOUR FREE LEG SIDE.
THEN TURN BACK TOWARDS THE FABRIC.

PLACE YOUR FOOT AGAINST THE FAR PIECE OF FABRIC.
BE SURE TO GO ABOVE THE CLOSER PIECE AND NOT UNDER.

AS YOU ROLL UP AND INTO THE FABRIC, BE SURE TO PUSH THE 'FAR' PIECE OF FABRIC DOWN TO THE ANKLE WITH YOUR FREE FOOT. OTHERWISE THE FABRIC STAYS HIGH ON THE KNEE AND CAN BE PAINFUL.

TO EXIT

Hold the fabric high above your head and unwind back the way you came - unwind slowly to avoid whiplash - try to keep your body as upright as possible as if you are standing up straight.

LIBERTY LEAN

ENTRY

From a single footlock, bend and raise your free knee so your thigh is parallel to the floor.

Place the fabric deep into the pocket of your free legs hip crease.

Keep your free knee raised high and bent while you begin to lean in the opposite direction. (if left leg is bent and raised then lean right)

As you lean over, fold your body in half as if you were trying to touch your nose to your knee. (the crunching motion of folding helps you to keep your balance).

SAFETY CONCERNS

If you do not have a solid 'nose to knee' fold you will fall back out of the balance.

TECHNIQUES / TIPS

Keep your supporting leg straight.

It will be slightly painful but you must keep the fabric deep into your hip / thigh crease to have the proper balance.

If you are having trouble letting go once in position fold your chest to your thigh even more (nose to knee) .

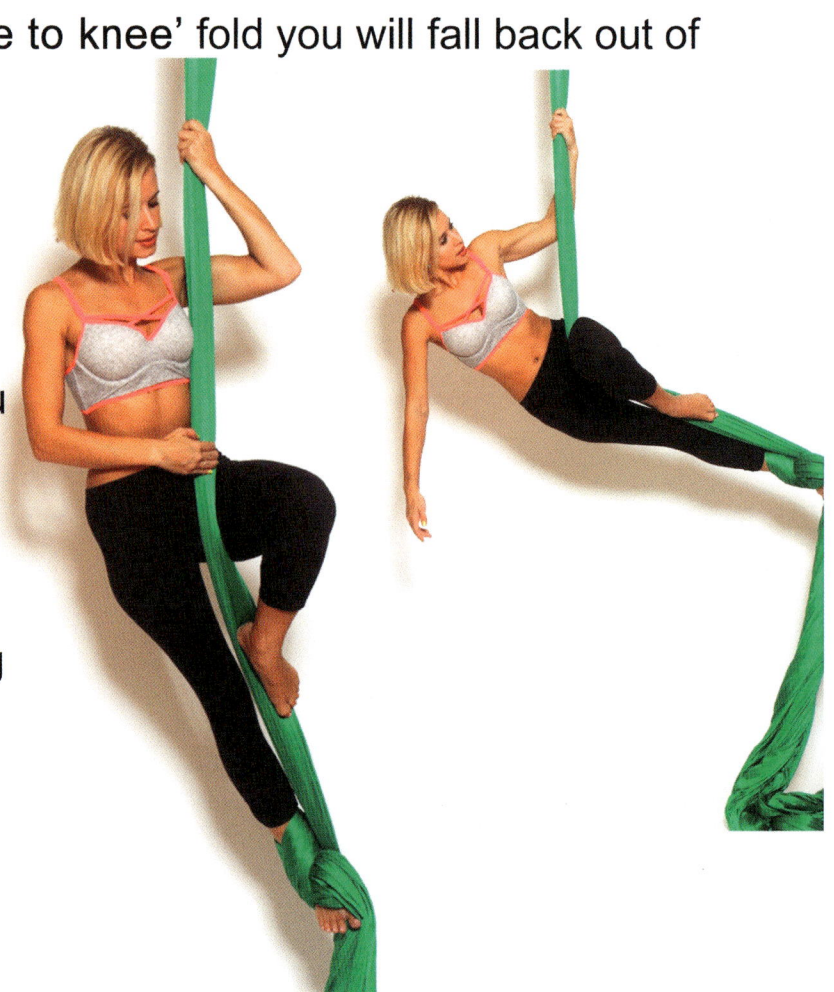

COCOON

ENTRY
From a single footlock, split the two pieces and turn sideways into the fabric so that one piece is at your chest and the other against your back.

Lean your weight into the 'front' piece and squeeze the fabric in between your neck and shoulder for balance. Reach your hands low behind your booty and begin to spread out the fabric behind you.

Once the fabric is spread lean your booty back into the fabric and begin to squat down.

SAFETY CONCERNS
Balance - be sure to have the fabric snug between your neck and shoulders while opening the back piece.

TECHNIQUES/ TIPS
It is common for your footlock to come undone while seated depending on the angle of your foot. Generally you won't fall out, you will just have a tight wrap to deal with when you want to come out.

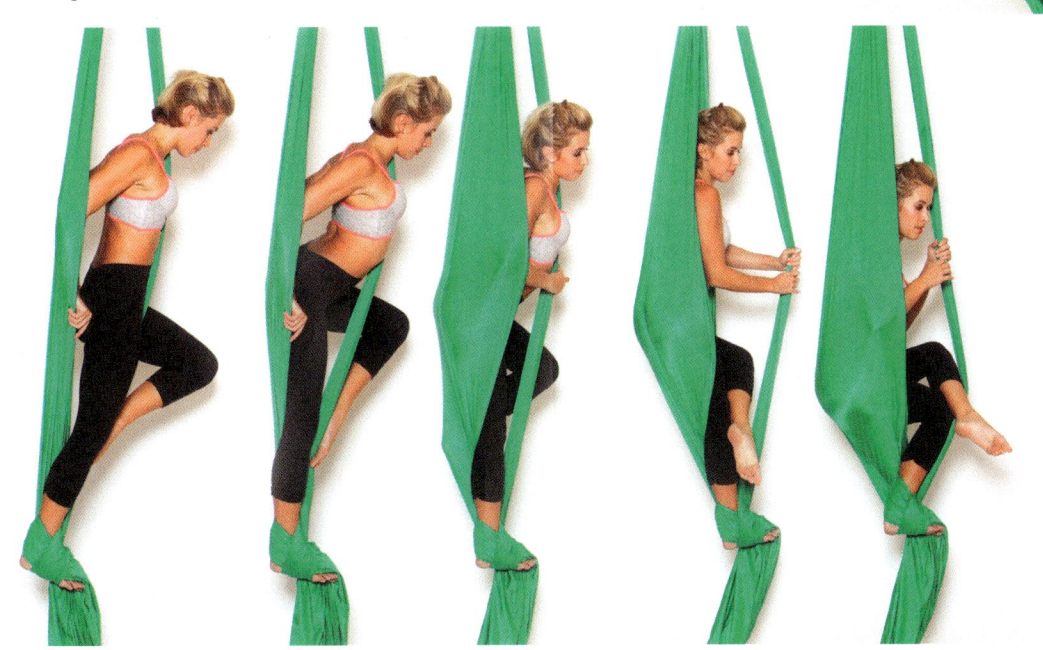

PG 35

MAN IN THE MOON

ENTRY
From a single footlock, split the fabric into two pieces and turn your body sideways in the fabric.
Lean your weight against the 'back' piece of fabric nestling the fabric against one shoulder.
Place your free foot against the 'front' piece hip level or higher.
Push the front piece of fabric away from the body while arching your back and driving your hips up to the ceiling.
(the trick with this is not to place any weight on your locked foot but to distribute your weight against your shoulder and free foot)

SAFETY CONCERNS
Watch your balance as its easy to tilt off to one side here.

TECHNIQUES / TIPS
Most people have problems with this because they continue to try to 'stand' on their locked foot. bend your locked leg as you lift up your hips to release any tension on it.

If you find you have a solid hold here you can straighten both arms out by your ears... this balance takes practice so be careful.

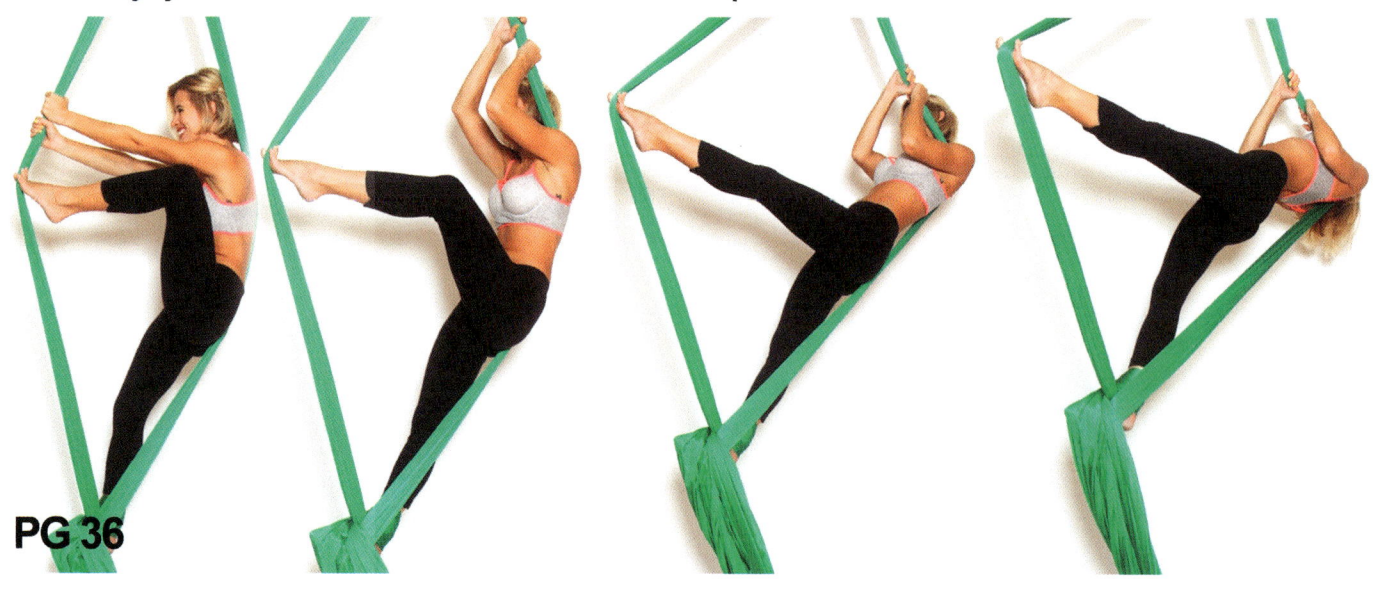

TO EXIT
Slowly lower your body back down - sometimes the fabric can slip off your foot and snap back.

CLOTHESLINE

ENTRY
From a single footlock, bend / raise your free leg high and hook the your 'knee pit' over the fabric.
Grab tightly onto your ankle and begin to lower your chest down to the floor.

TO EXIT
Reach your hand up for the fabric and pull your chest back up.

SAFETY CONCERNS
Be careful not to lose grip on your ankle as you will slip off.

Getting back up takes alot of core strength so practice low first.

TECHNIQUES / TIPS
Keep your locked leg as straight as possible.

Treat your high knee as a pivot point carrying most of the weight on your knee while pushing out through the other leg.

Keep as much distance as possible between your high knee and locked foot.

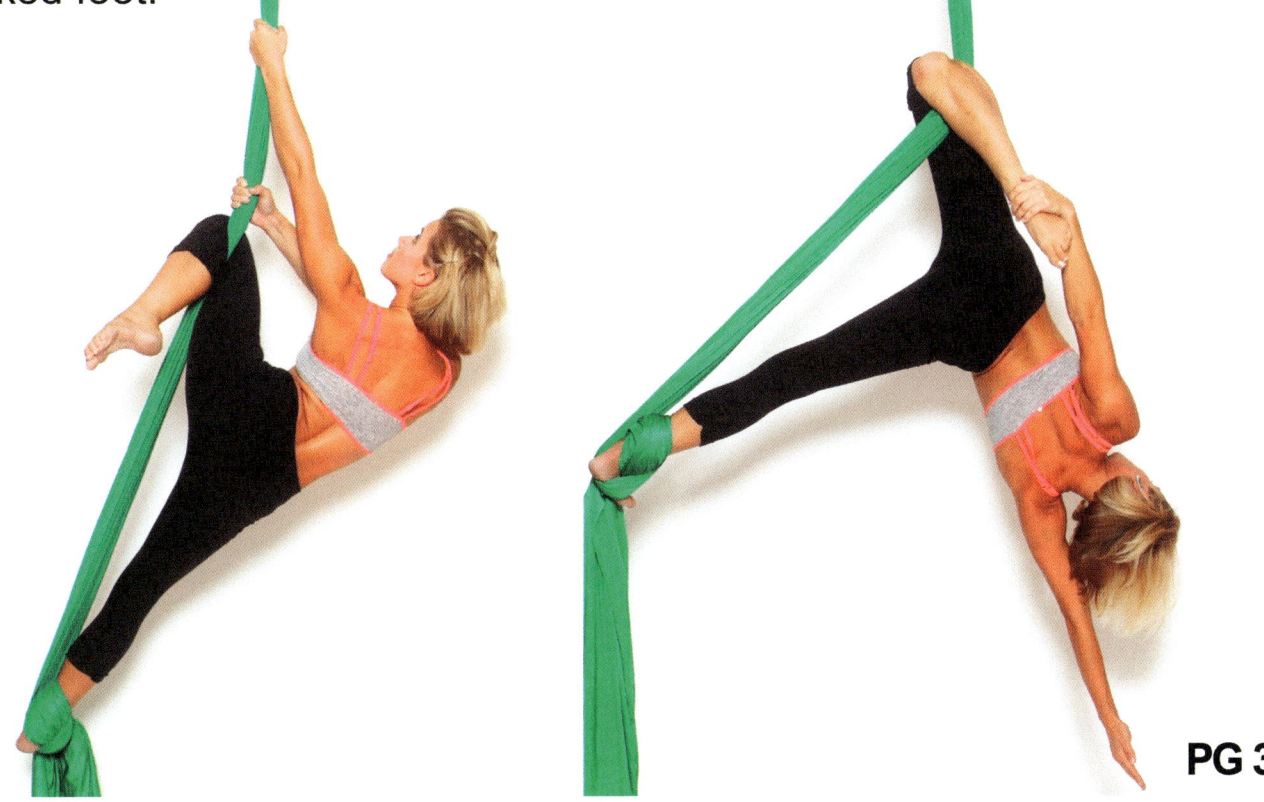

PG 37

360 TWIST

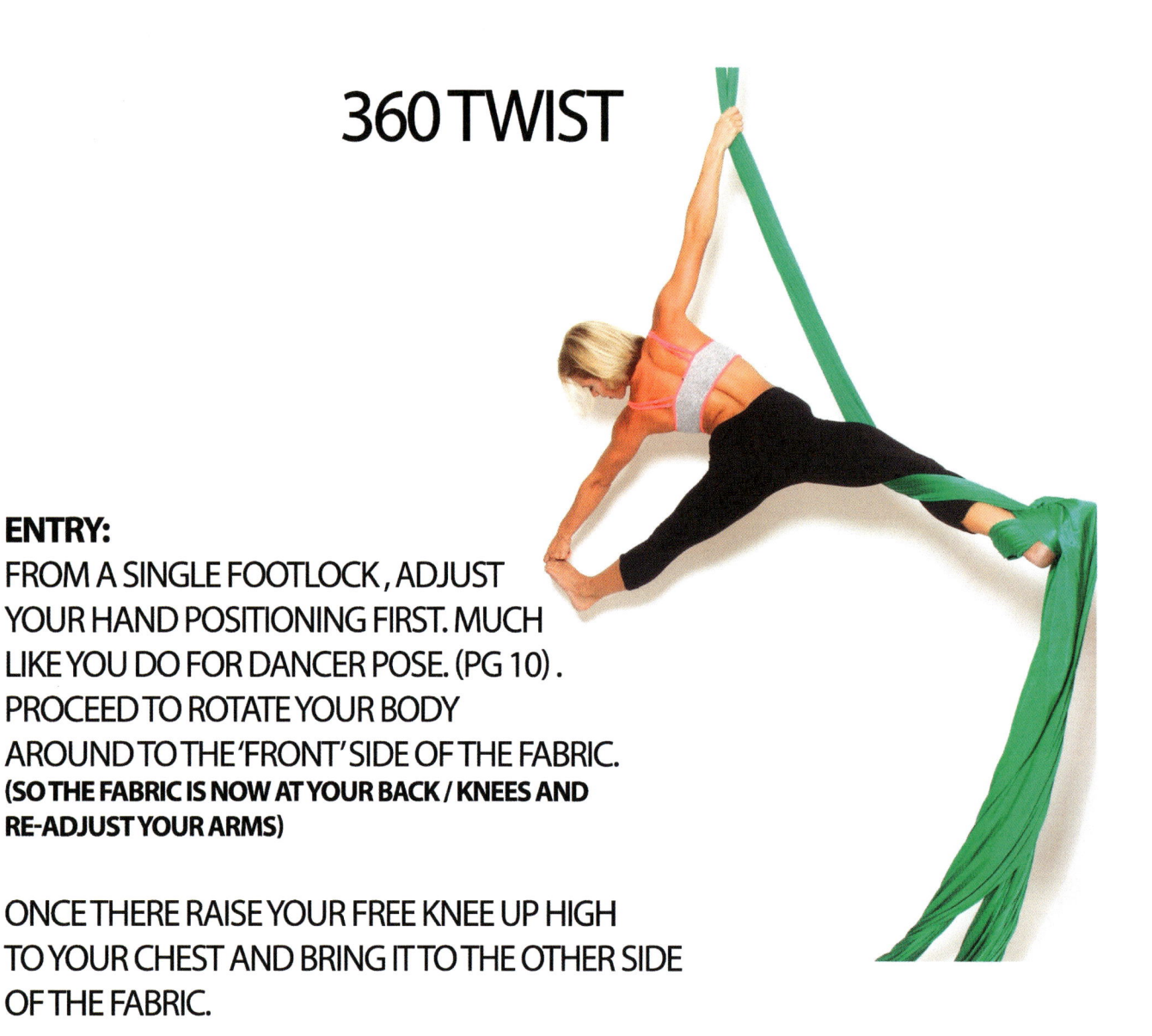

ENTRY:
FROM A SINGLE FOOTLOCK, ADJUST YOUR HAND POSITIONING FIRST. MUCH LIKE YOU DO FOR DANCER POSE. (PG 10). PROCEED TO ROTATE YOUR BODY AROUND TO THE 'FRONT' SIDE OF THE FABRIC. **(SO THE FABRIC IS NOW AT YOUR BACK / KNEES AND RE-ADJUST YOUR ARMS)**

ONCE THERE RAISE YOUR FREE KNEE UP HIGH TO YOUR CHEST AND BRING IT TO THE OTHER SIDE OF THE FABRIC.

FROM THERE, STICK YOUR FREE LEG OUT TO THE SIDE AND LEAN YOUR BODY IN THAT DIRECTION. **TO EXIT** - BRING YOUR FREE KNEE BACK TO ITS ORIGINAL SIDE AND UNWIND YOUR BODY AROUND THE FABRIC.

SAFETY CONCERNS:
ITS EASY TO LOSE GRIP ON THE FABRIC SO BE MINDFUL OF THIS.

TECHNIQUES / TIPS:
HOLD HANDS HIGH ABOVE YOUR HEAD AND ADJUST THEM FIRST BEFORE TRYING TO ADJUST YOUR BODY.

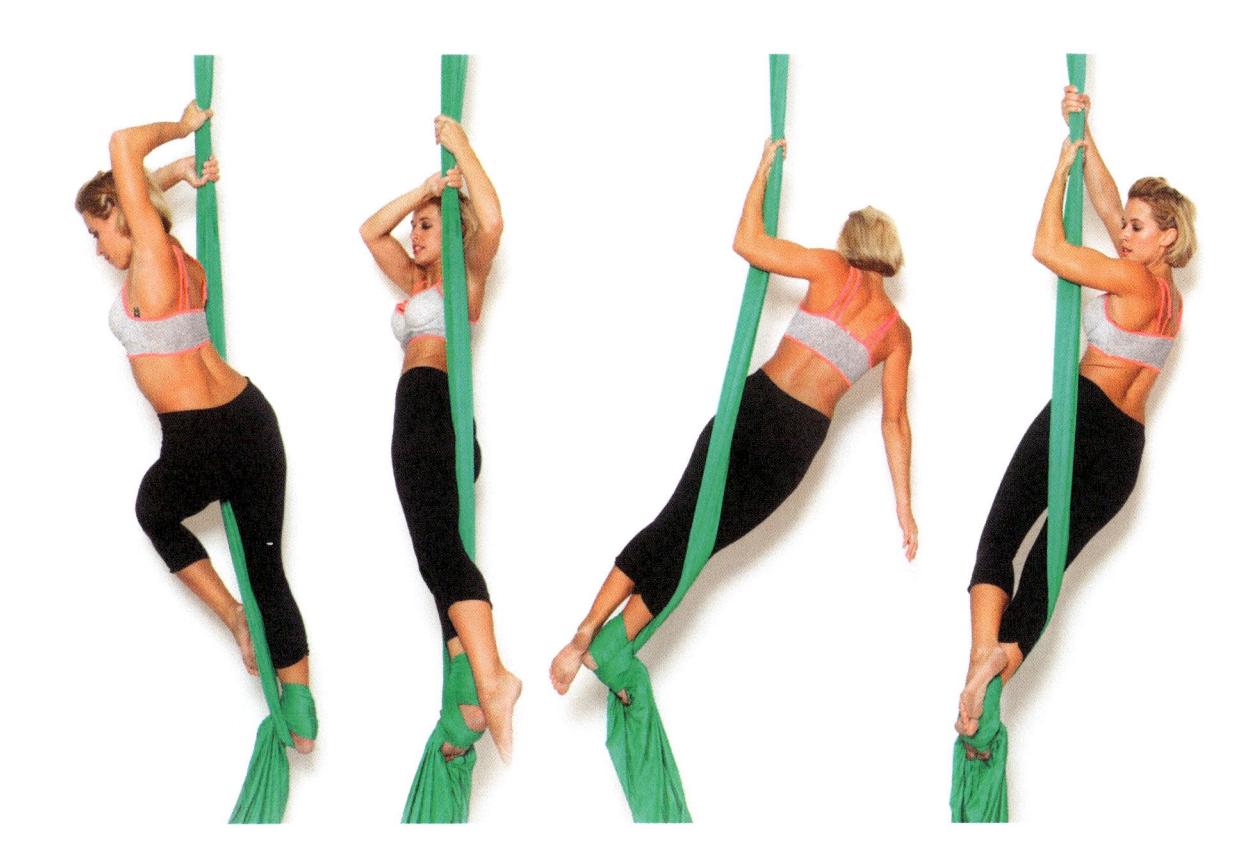

If the left foot is free, you will be going initially 'left' as you twist around.

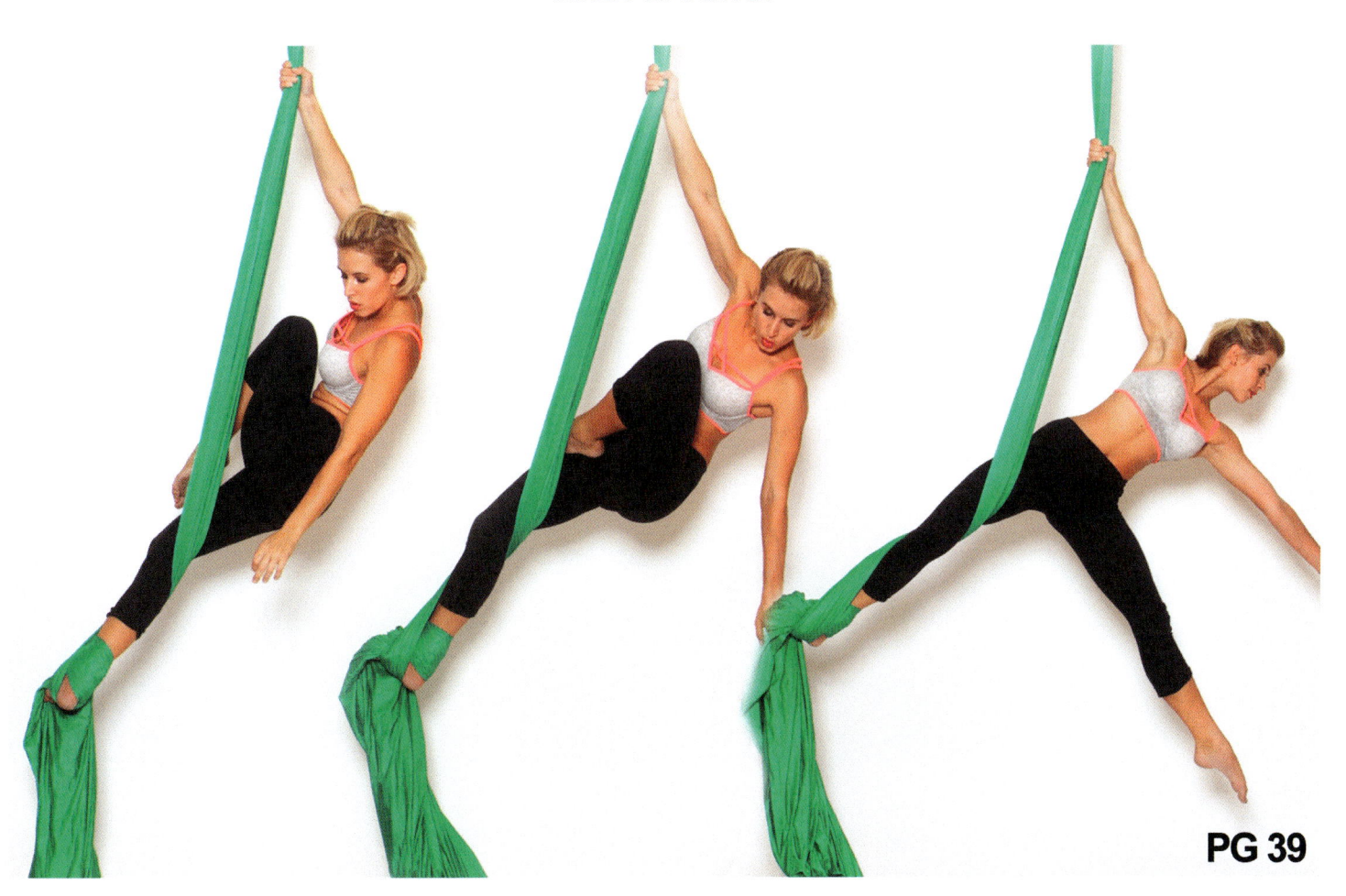

PG 39

MARIONETTE

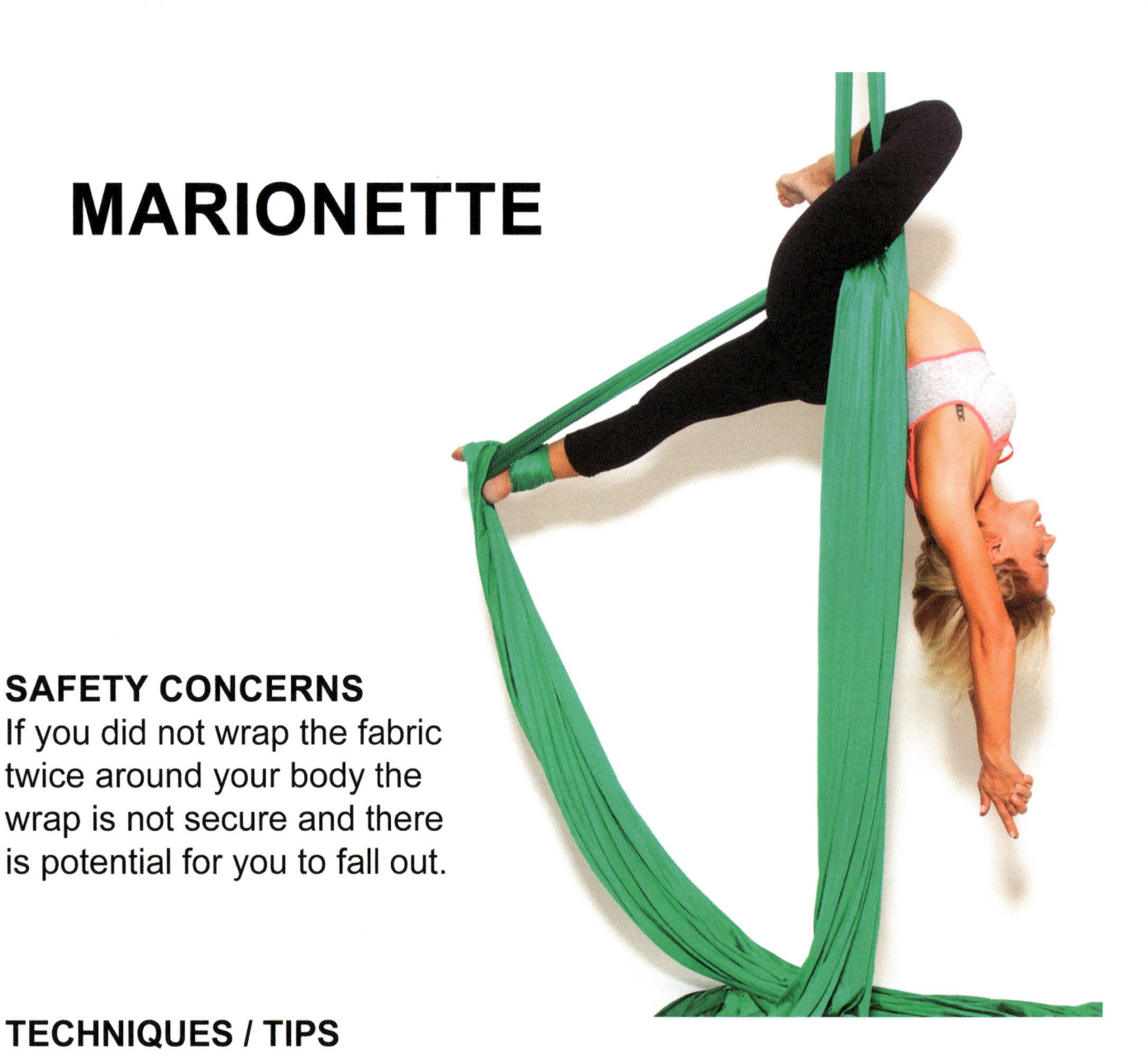

SAFETY CONCERNS
If you did not wrap the fabric twice around your body the wrap is not secure and there is potential for you to fall out.

TECHNIQUES / TIPS
Remember you must have the free piece tucked into your armpit before wrapping around the body.
(if the free piece is the left piece then it tucks into the left armpit)

The fabric can be hard to wrap around so use your free knee (**bent and raised**) to help keep the fabric from falling down the body.

You can do this pose with only one wrap around the bady ..
However you must hold on tightly to the tail of your fabric ...
Letting go of this piece could cause you to fall out.

ENTRY

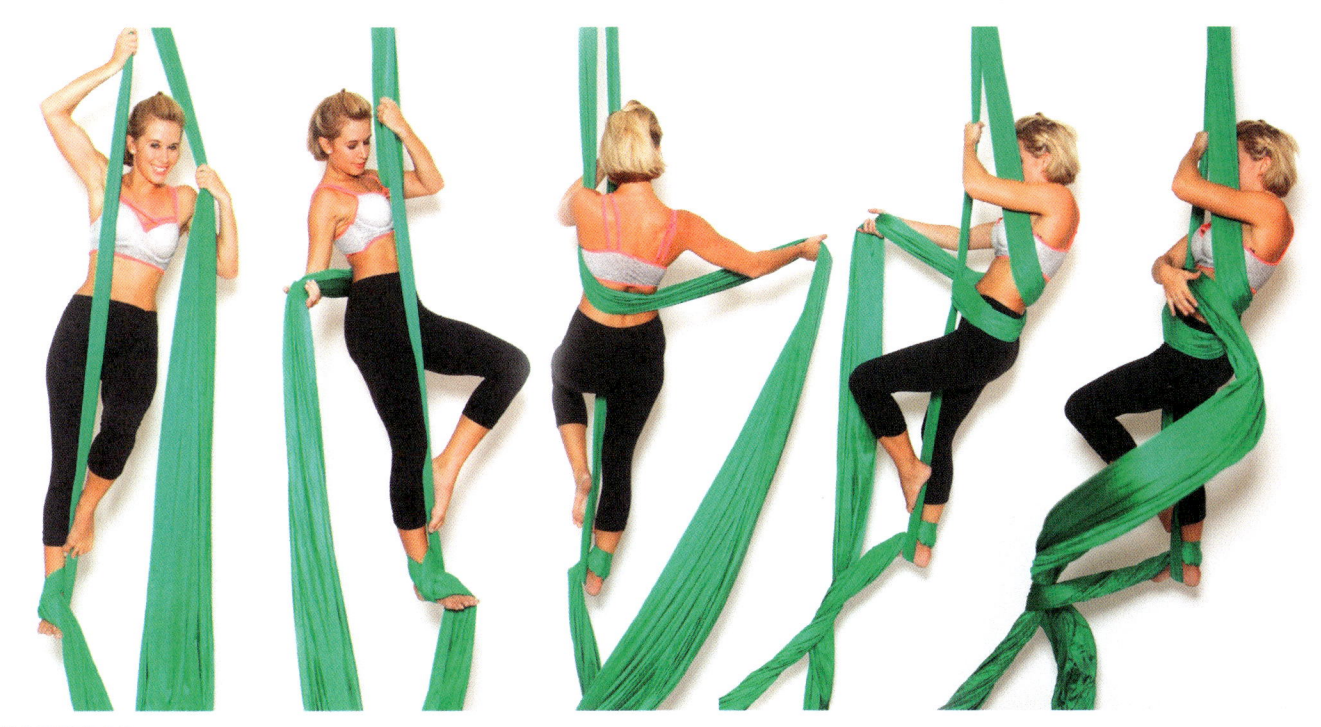

Split the fabric into two pieces and do a single footlock on just one piece.

Tuck the other piece of fabric in your armpit and begin to wrap that piece around your body two times. (If you keep your free leg bent and raised high it will help to keep the fabric from falling down while you are wrapping)

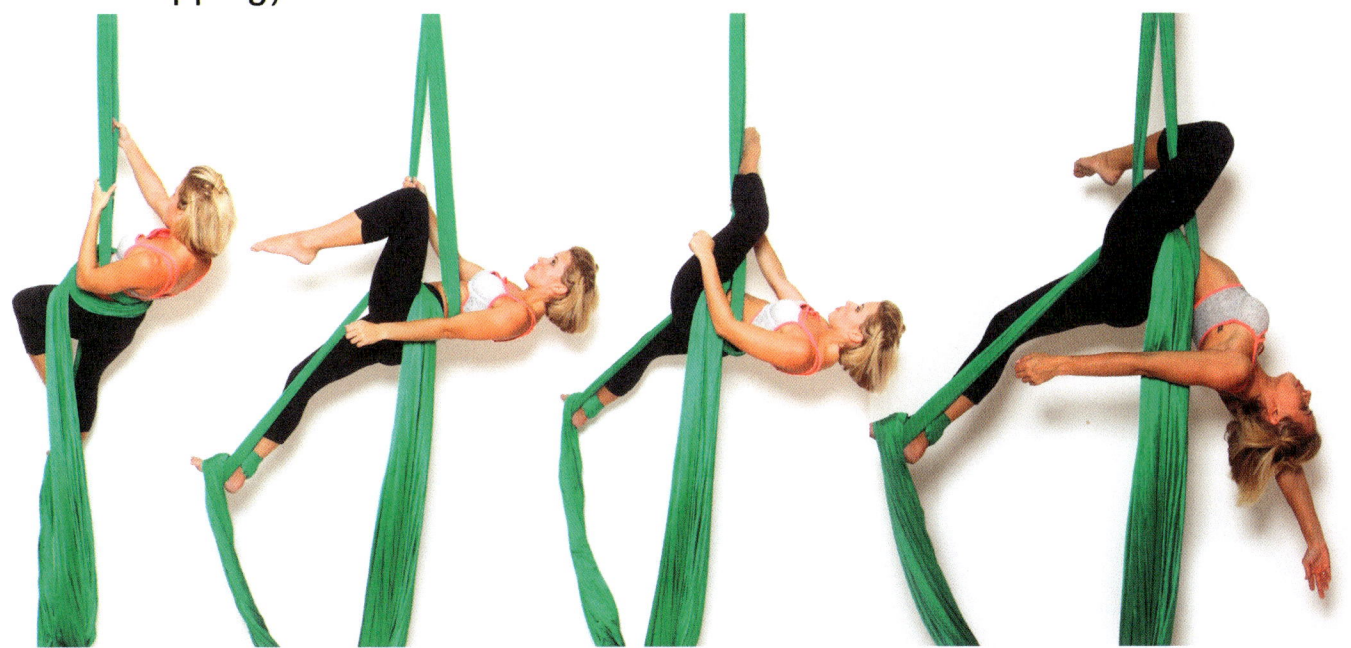

Once you've wrapped the fabric two times lean back and begin to hook your free leg up over both pieces of fabric.

TO EXIT - unhook your top leg, stand back up and unravel the free piece of fabric,

PG 41

MARIONETTE INTO DANCER

ENTRY
From marionette, hook your top leg in between the two fabric pieces. As you go into dancer you will be turning in the direction of your locked foot (right foot locked turn right and vice versa)

Hold onto to the right piece (or left if left foot is locked) with both hands and begin to pull your body up and in between the two pieces.

You want your chest resting against the 'front' piece of fabric.

SAFETY CONCERNS
This requires alot of flexibility and can be a bigger stretch than it looks ... so stretch first.

TECHNIQUES / TIPS
Hold both hands on one piece as you rotate in.

Try to pull yourself up high above the fabric, then turn your body and then drop your weight back into the fabric.

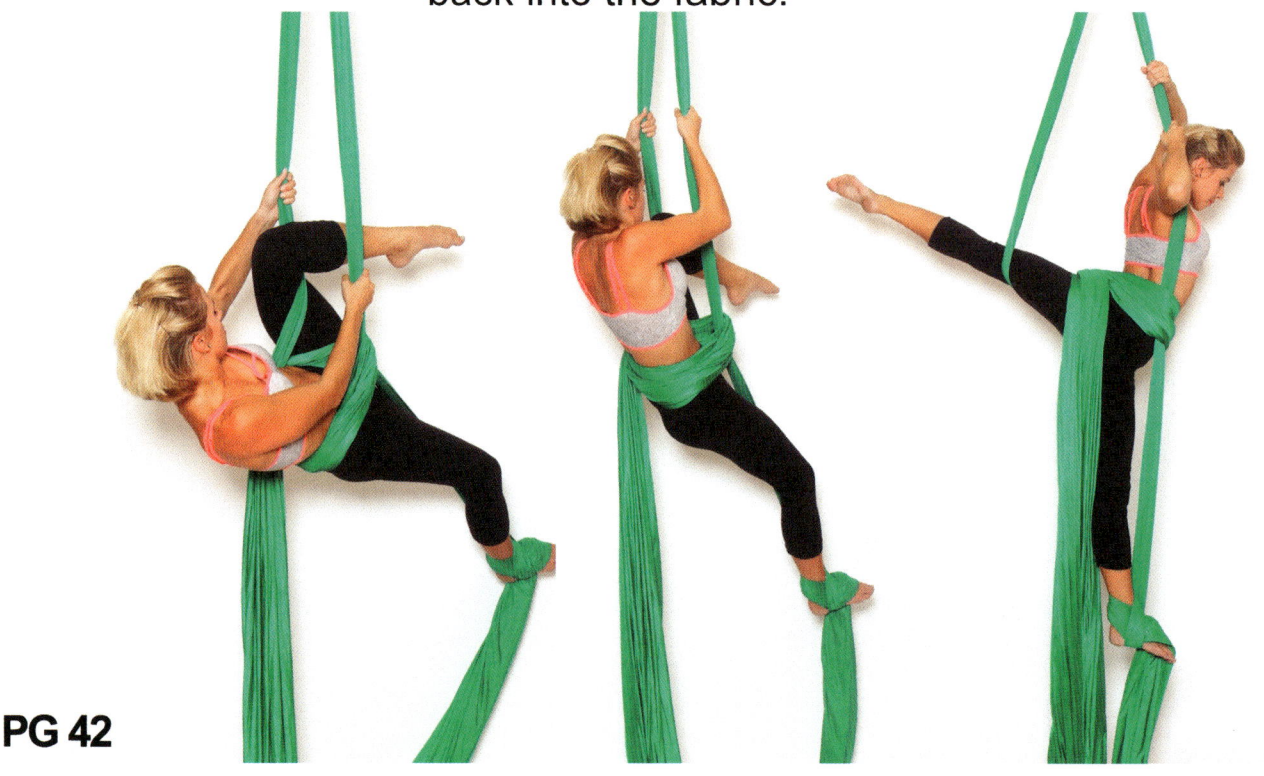

FLAG

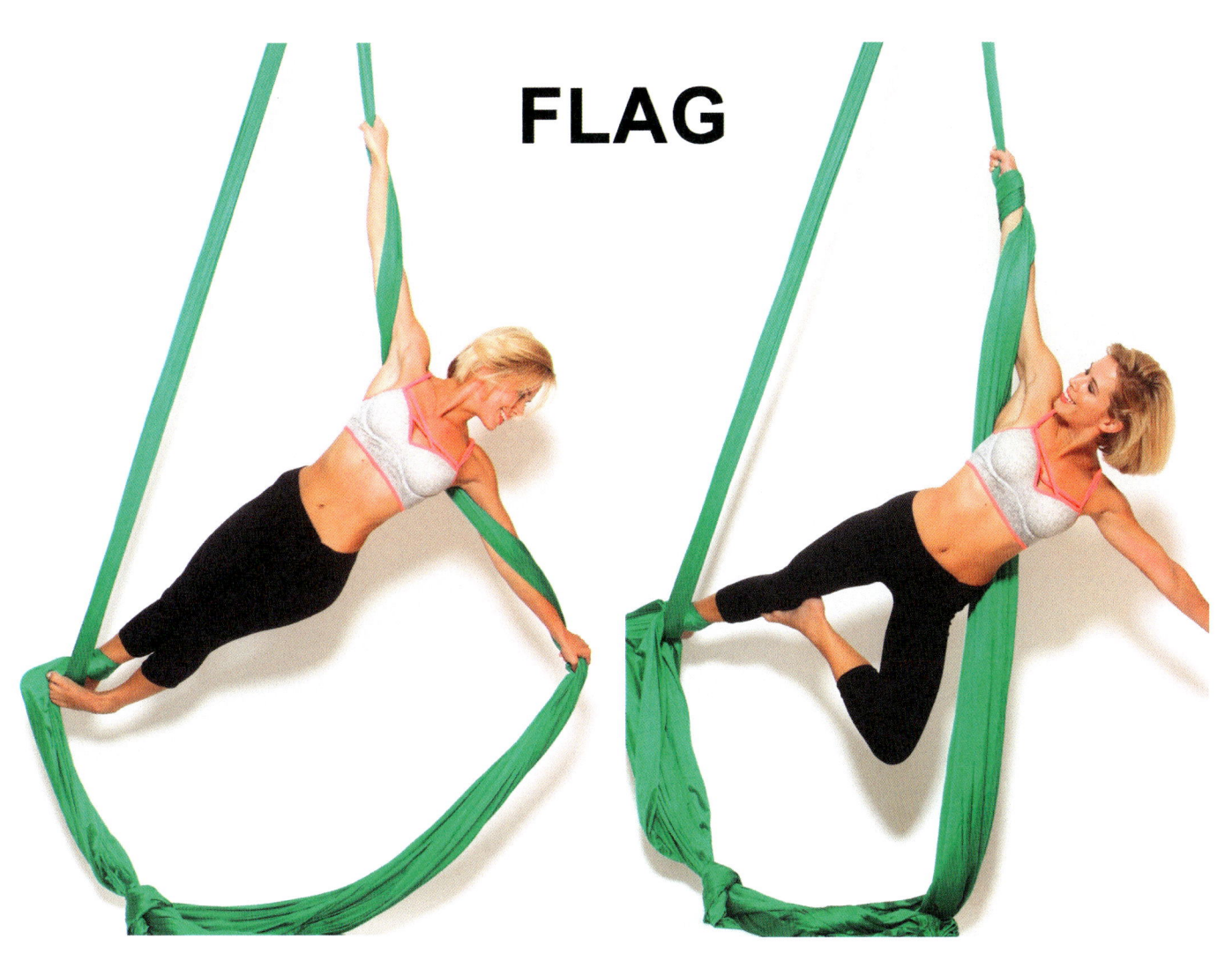

Entry on the next page . . . (pg 44)

SAFETY CONCERNS
Balance and Grip

TECHNIQUES / TIPS
The free fabric should not be carrying any of your weight before you begin to wrap your top arm.

Fabric should run along the armpit and shoulder blades.... not the neck!

This can also be done with just a single wrist wrap / one arm. This requires more grip strength.

ENTRY
Split the fabric into two pieces and do a single footlock on just one piece.
(same side arm will be high so if your right foot is locked then your right hand will be high)

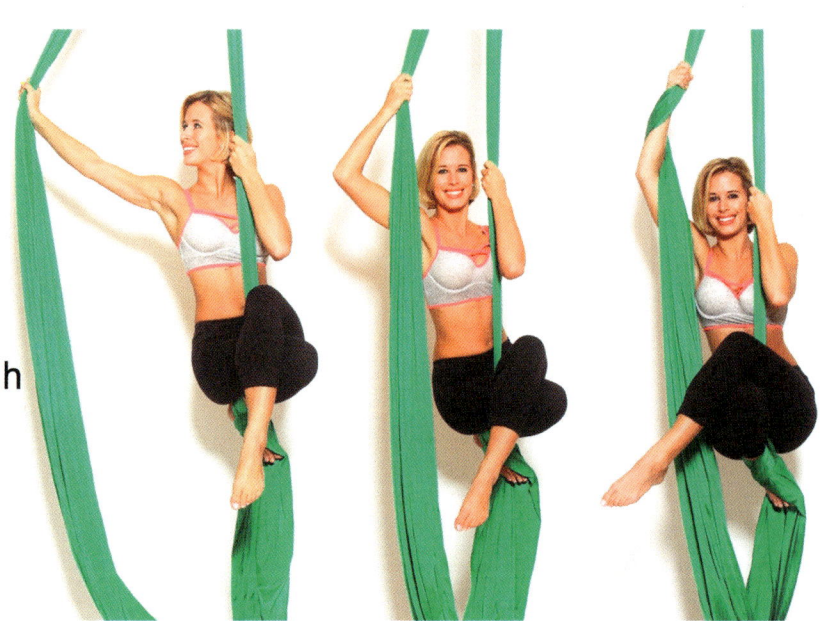

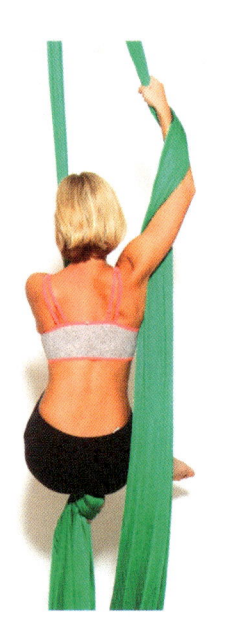

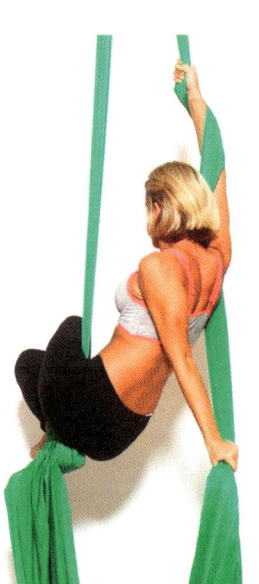

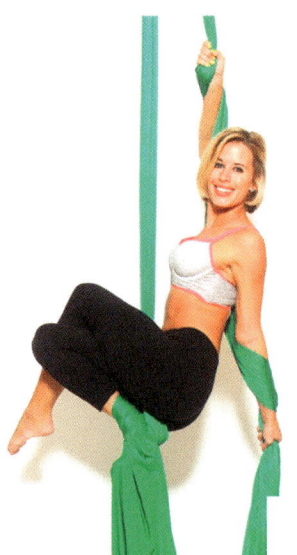

Reach your same side arm up and wrap it around the free fabric ... Get a good grip and then wrap your bottom arm low around the fabric.

Note in the pic how the farbic is running along the inside of her armpit. This makes the hold more secure... If you find the fabric is hitting the back of your neck you're not quite right and should re - wrap your arms.

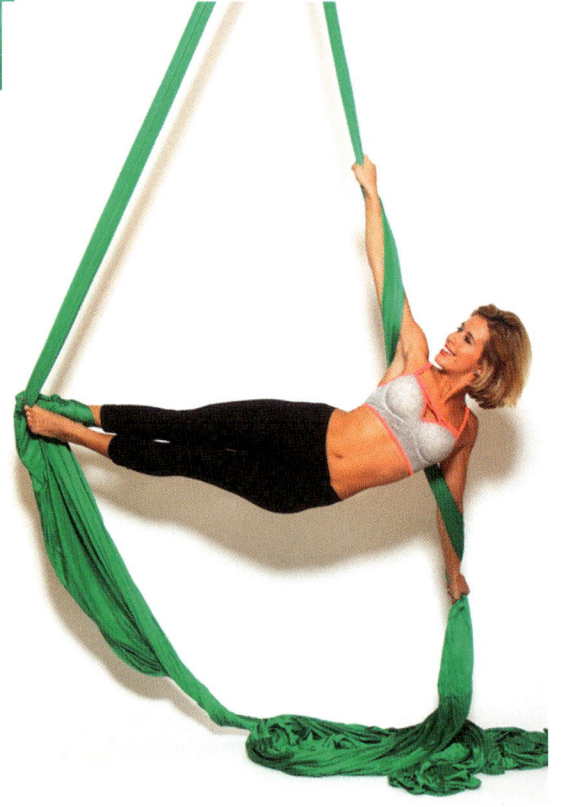

LADYSIT HANG

ENTRY
From your LadySit pose (pg 3), cross your top leg in as much as possible and grab tightly onto your ankle.
Slowly begin to lower yourself backwards. The fabric should be running across the top thigh and just slightly under the top knee.

TO EXIT
Do a big sit up to reach back up for the fabric.

SAFETY CONCERNS
This is very intense on the hips so stretch yourself out first.

The cross in the top leg is your safety, if your leg uncrosses you fall out.

TECHNIQUES / TIPS
Some students have a problem keeping their thighs close together, you do not want your knees to spread away from each other so cross your legs tightly!
(imagine you really 'gotta go' :P)

This pose can be done without holding on to the ankle but you must be very careful and very aware of your top leg. Again, if your top leg uncrosses... You fall out!

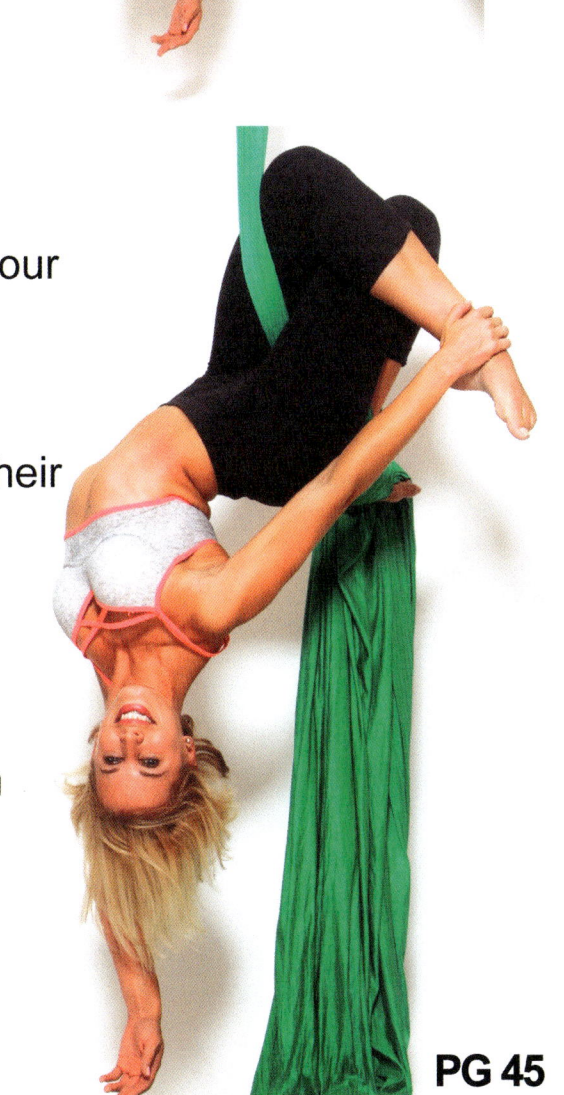

LOTUS HANG

ENTRY
Very similar to a ladysit, but as you begin to squat down place the top of your free foot directly underneath the knee pit of the opposite leg. (Make sure the fabric is still in between both legs)

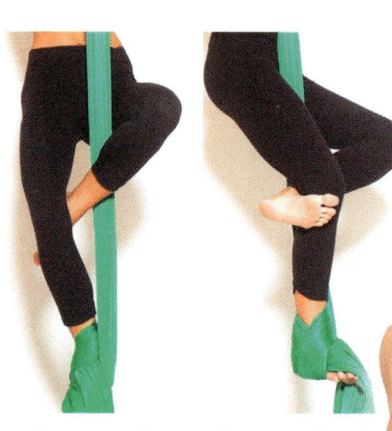

As you begin to squat and once you have placed your foot correctly ... Allow your knees to widen and point away from each other. Be sure to keep your 'top' foot directly in the knee pit of the other leg.

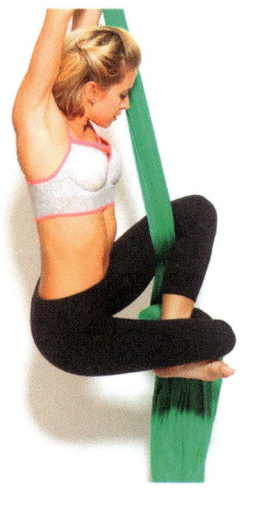

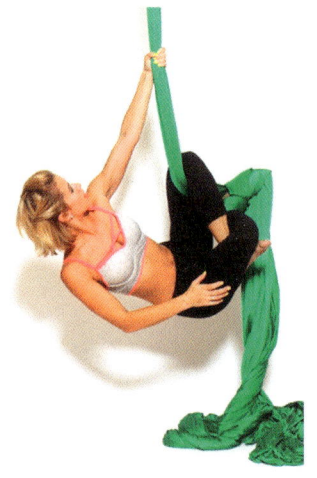

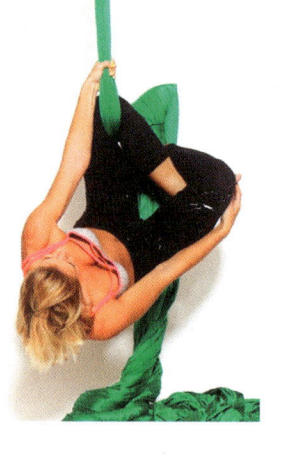

As you lean back to go upside down the fabric should be under the free knee.... Or under the knee of the top leg.

SAFETY CONCERNS
Make sure the free foot is tucked under the opposite knee.

This is a huge stretch for the hips so lower down slowly!

TECHNIQUES / TIPS
Knees should be wide and pointing away from each other.

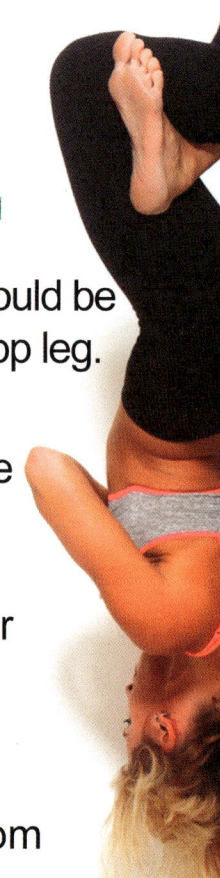

PG 46

CHAPTER 5
DOUBLE FOOTLOCK POSES - SPLITS

ENTRY
From a double footlock, gently split the legs open and allow the body to sink down low.

If doing a right or left side split . . . turn your hips so they face the appropriate side.

If doing middle ... Keep your hips facing forward and tops of the feet facing upwards.

SAFTEY CONCERNS
It is very easy to sink down too fast and pull a muscle.
Be warmed up and go slowly.

TECHNIQUES / TIPS
You can hold onto both pieces with your hands ...
Or hold both hands on one single piece.

If you have a solid grip you can hold with just one hand.

To have the illusion of an oversplit ... Make one footlock significantly higher than the other.

SPLIT ROLL UP

ENTRY

Choose either a left or right side split. If left ... Then you will be turning left and vice versa ...

Hold onto the 'front' piece with both hands. Look in the direction you want to rotate and begin to turn your body in that direction. (follow with your body where your eyes are looking) ...

As you look and rotate in the appropriate direction ... Bring your front foot around to the inside of the fabrics and then back to the front to a regular split again.

SAFETY CONCERNS

It is possible to lose the lock on your front foot as you wrap around so be mindful of this.

TECHNIQUES / TIPS

In order to not lose the lock on your front foot keep as much tension on the fabric as possible between your hands and your front foot.

Generally two rolls is good ... Three if you are very flexible.

As you roll your back leg will begin to elevate higher than your front foot.

PG 49

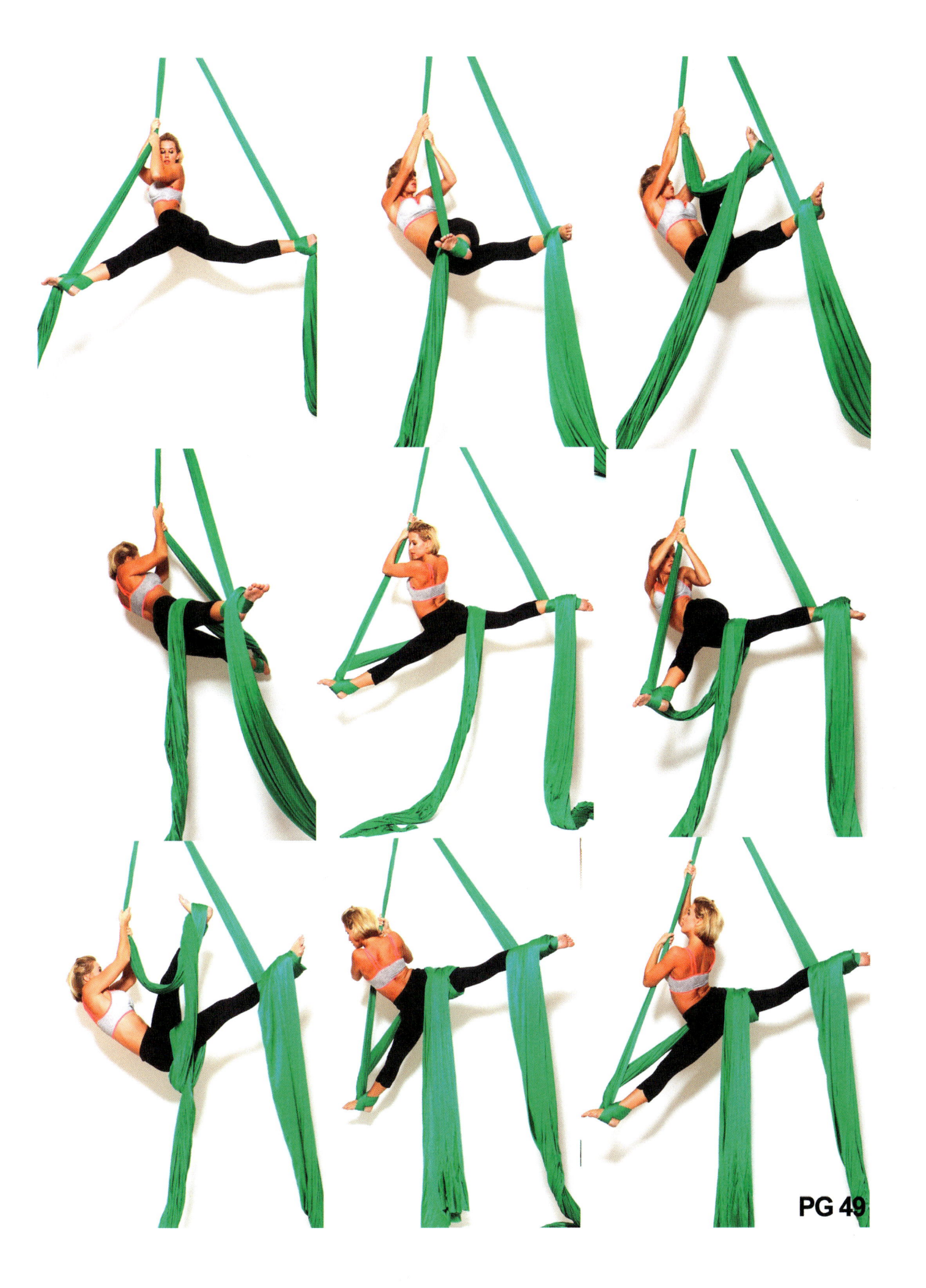

CUPID SEAT

ENTRY
From a double footlock, turn your body sideways so that one piece is in front and the other at your back. Keep the back piece resting against your booty and bring your back leg forward. Cross your back leg over the top of your front silk, bend the top knee and rest your weight into the back piece of fabric.

SAFETY CONCERNS
The back piece of fabric must stay in the middle of your booty in order for you to sit back.

TECHNIQUES / TIPS
Cross your back leg over just like a guy would cross his legs.. ankle over knee.

Make sure your hooking your back leg over the actual silks, not just the knee.

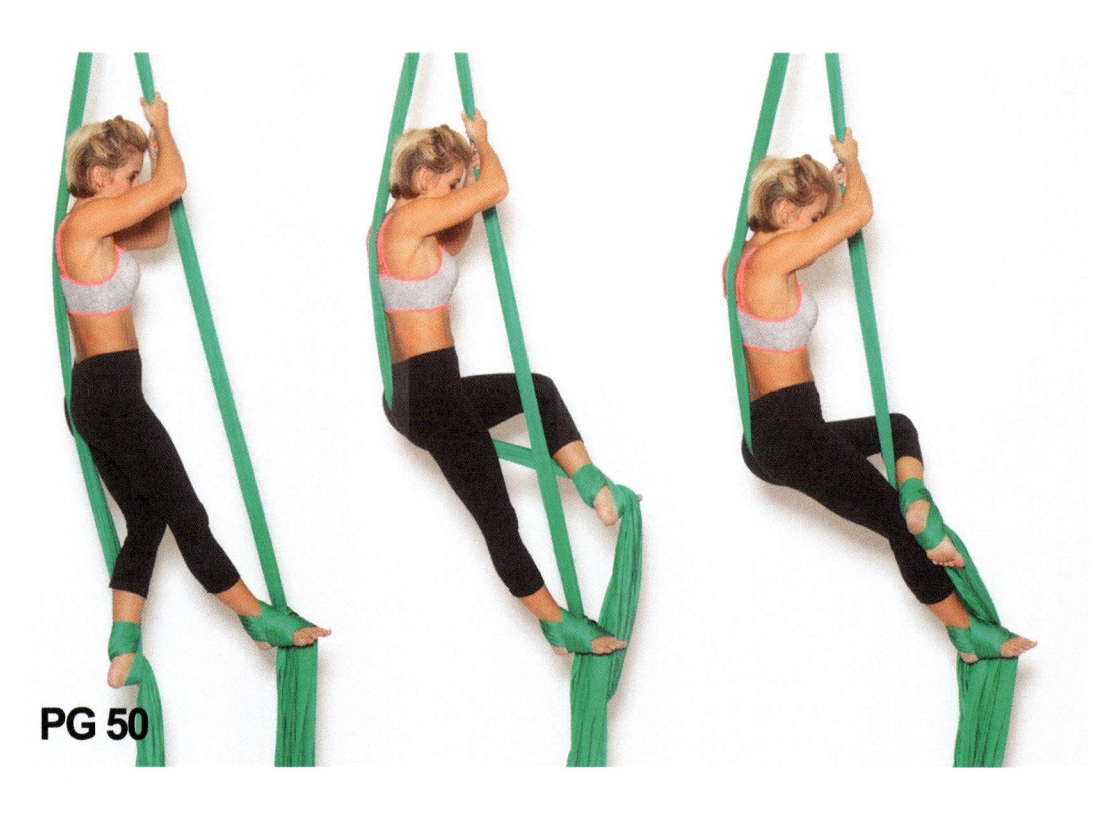

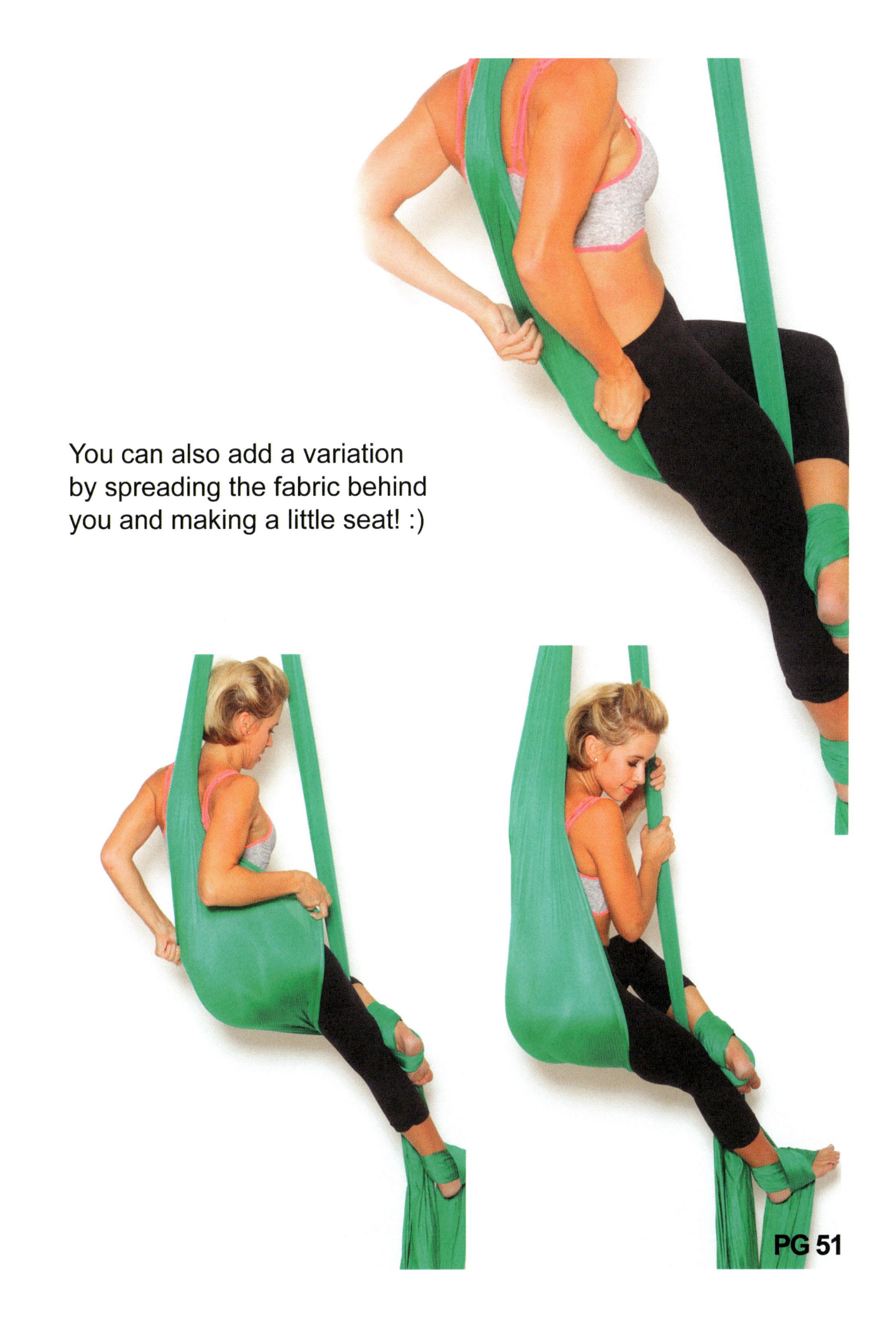

You can also add a variation by spreading the fabric behind you and making a little seat! :)

CROSSBACK STRADDLE

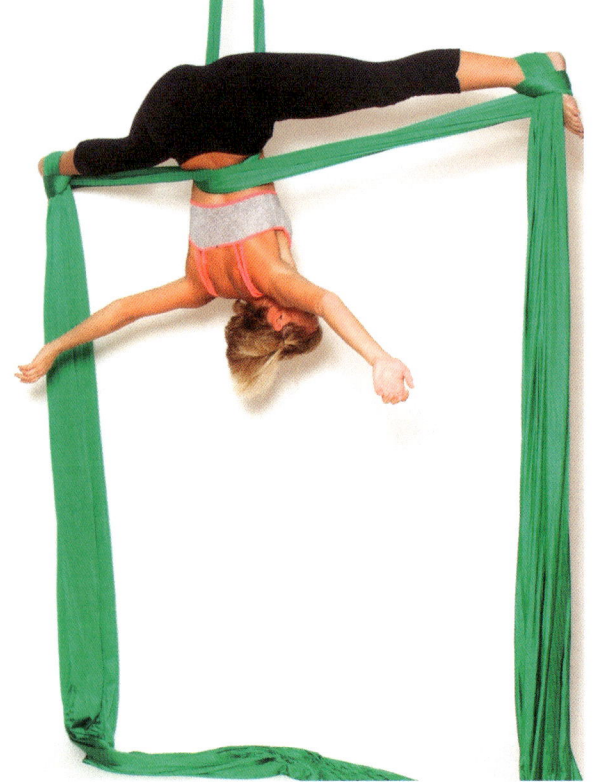

ENTRY
From a double footlock ...
Bring your legs together and your body through to the front side of the fabric.
(so that both pieces of fabric are at your back)

From here ... adjust your hand positioning...
One hand reaches behind both pieces to grab the opposite fabric ...
The other hand stays on the front of the fabric and grabs the opposite piece ...

Then you must pull the pieces across each other and set your shoulders between them.

(to do this successfully you must keep your legs together and your booty on the front side of the fabric)

NOTE
Once you set the shoulders in ... Bring the arms through as well.

Once the arms are through ... Straddle the legs as wide as you can so the fabric forms an 'X' at your lower back. Keep your legs straight and wide and drive your toes up towards the ceiling. While doing so pull your body up with your arms (like a pull up) and then push against the fabric so that you start to pivot over the fabric and go upside down.

SAFTEY CONCERNS
Be sure to keep the 'X' at your lower back or you won't be able to get anywhere. (note the lower left pic)

TECHNIQUES / TIPS
Think of going back as a 3 step process ...
1 - straddle legs wide with toes up to ceiling
2 - pull up with arms and
3 - push back against the fabric.

The more you can pull up with your arms the easier it will be as this gives you more slack to get over.

TO EXIT
Reach up for the fabric by your inner thighs and rotate back to a standing position - carefully bring your shoulders back through the fabric ... carefully let the fabric uncross to its original position.

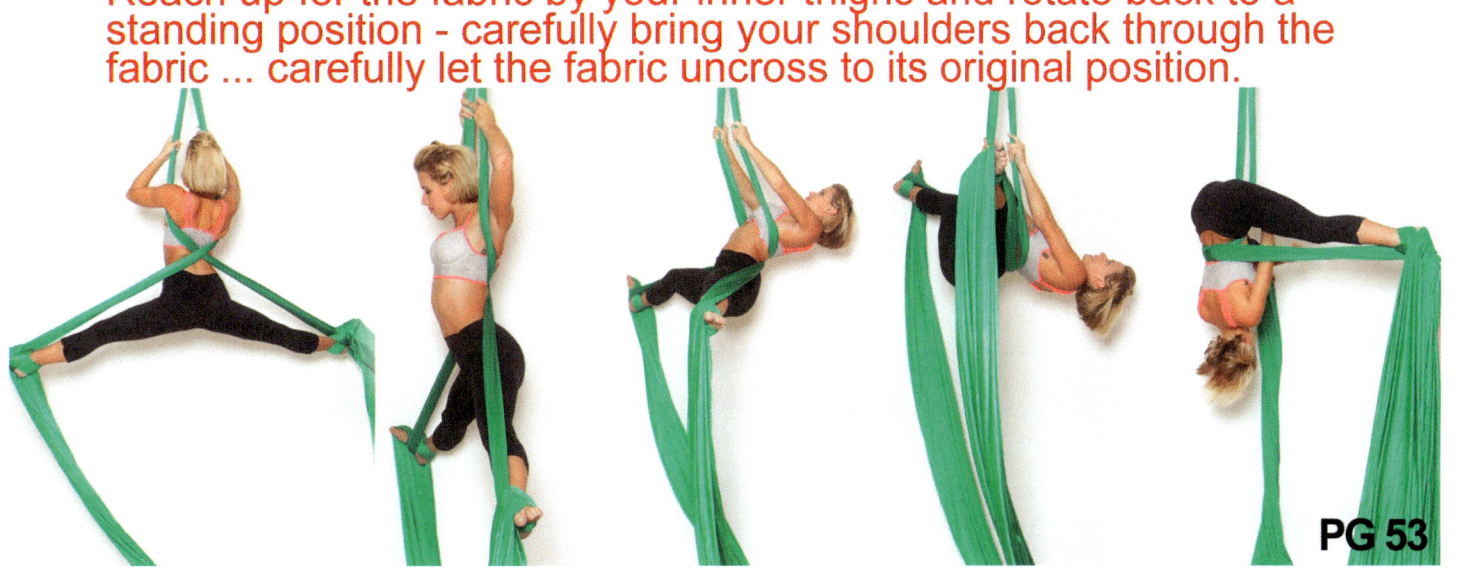

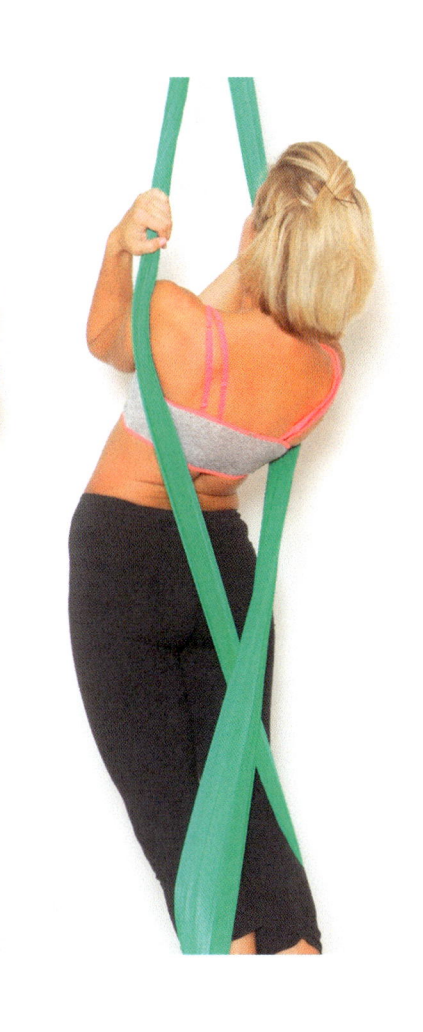

PG 53

CROSSBACK STRADDLE TO SPIDERMAN

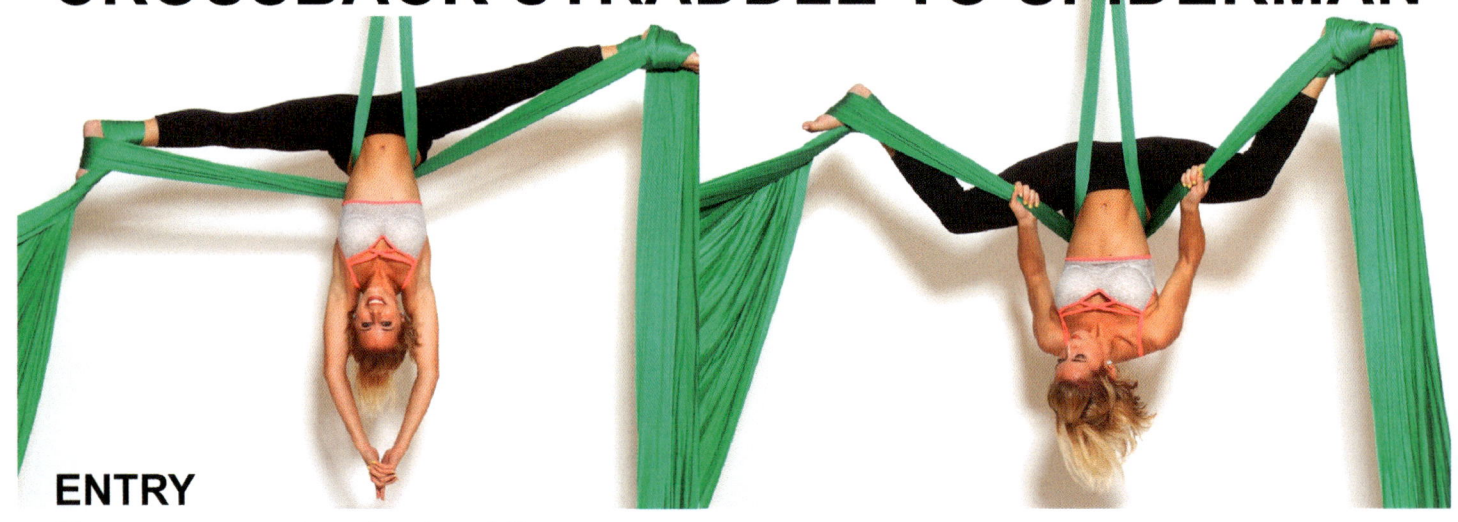

ENTRY
From a crossback straddle ...

Begin to bend your knees and allow the bottoms of your feet to come together.
(Note: you must have the fabric on the inside of your thighs as you bend your knees)

Your body will lower slightly, just relax and allow it to slide down the fabric.

SAFETY CONCERNS
The fabric running along side your legs MUST be against the inside of your thighs. If they are on the outside of your thighs against the booty, you will fall out!

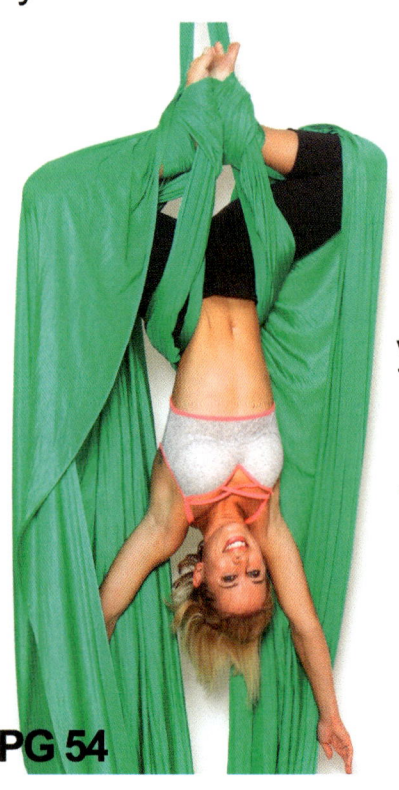

TECHNIQUES / TIPS
Use your hands to pull the fabric to the inside of your thighs as you bend your knees and sink down into the pose

Try to do both legs at the same time or you will end up lop-sided!

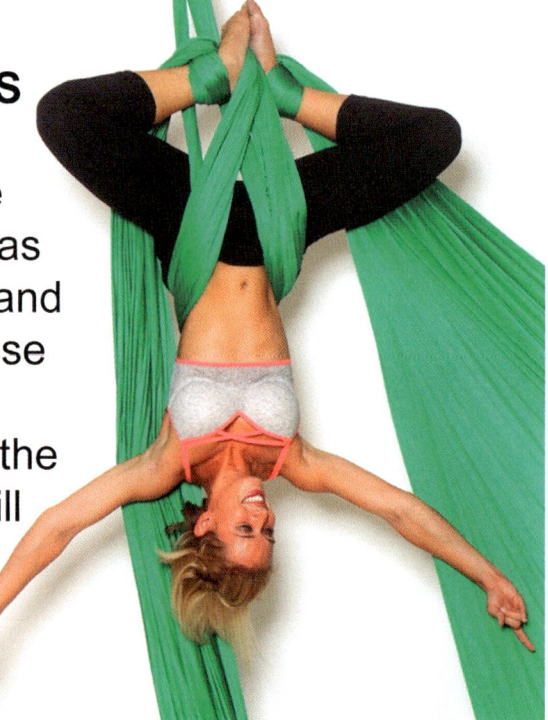

SPIDERMAN TO BUDDHA

ENTRY

From your spiderman ...
Open your feet so they can pass to the other side of the fabric and then bring them together again, as you do this rotate your body to an upright position and you're in your first Buddha!

In the first position the fabric is still crossed as an 'X' behind your back. Keep your feet together and legs in the same position ... Bring your upper body through to the front side of the fabric.

This will uncross the 'X' behind your back and sink you into a lower buddha from this second version you can reach up and stand straight up to exit.

SAFETY CONCERNS

The bottoms of your feet need to stay together except for when you are transitioning from spiderman to the first Buddha.

TECHNIQUES / TIPS

When in spiderman, you have to spread your feet apart first before you can rotate your body to an upright position.

Remember you won't be able to stand up until you have come to the second Buddha
(when your body/shoulders come through to the front of the fabric to release the 'X')

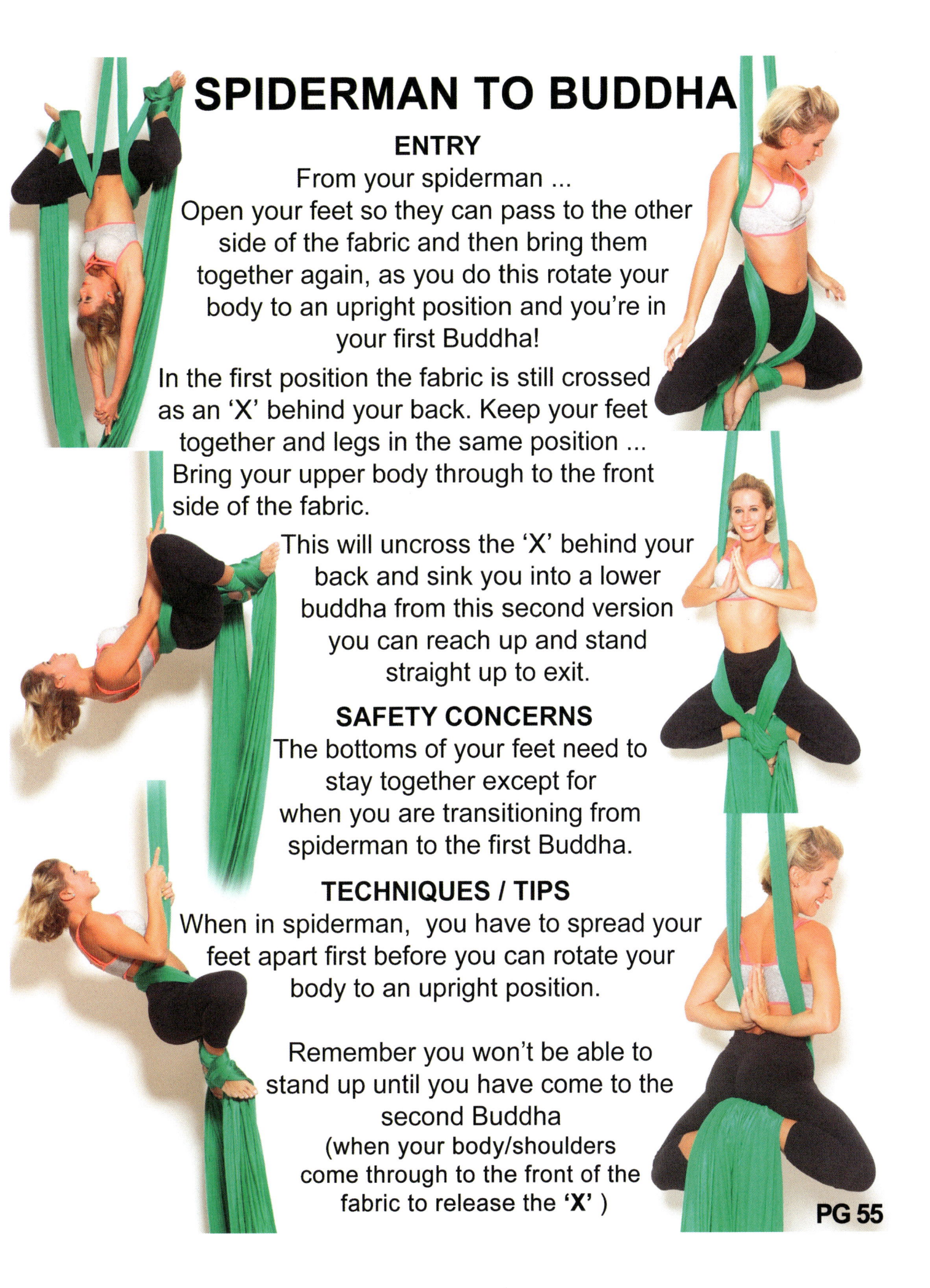

PG 55

"A windmill's true power is revealed only when it faces the wind; a person's only when he faces adversity." Zen Proverb

CHAPTER 6
INVERSIONS

Inversions are my personal favorite poses / tricks to practice; Inverting requires a deep sense of body awareness, it gives you the opportunity to approach and conquer possible fears.

Please note when working inversions, do so intelligently!

1. Practice with padding - place a mat / mattress or something very soft beneath you.

2. Perfect your trick low to the ground first.

3. Don't push yourself - if you feel like you are slipping .... YOU ARE! So come down!

4. Reserve some strength - its very easy to use up all of your strength getting into the pose and then find you have no strength left to exit the pose.

5. Don't panic - its easy to become disoriented and overwhelmed during your first inversions ... When that happens, take a breath and come down.

6. Patience is key - some students invert naturally... Whereas others may feel like it takes ages. Don't give up. your body will get used to the feeling and you will adjust as long as you keep at it!

7. Remember you are awesome! :)

INSIDE LEG HANG

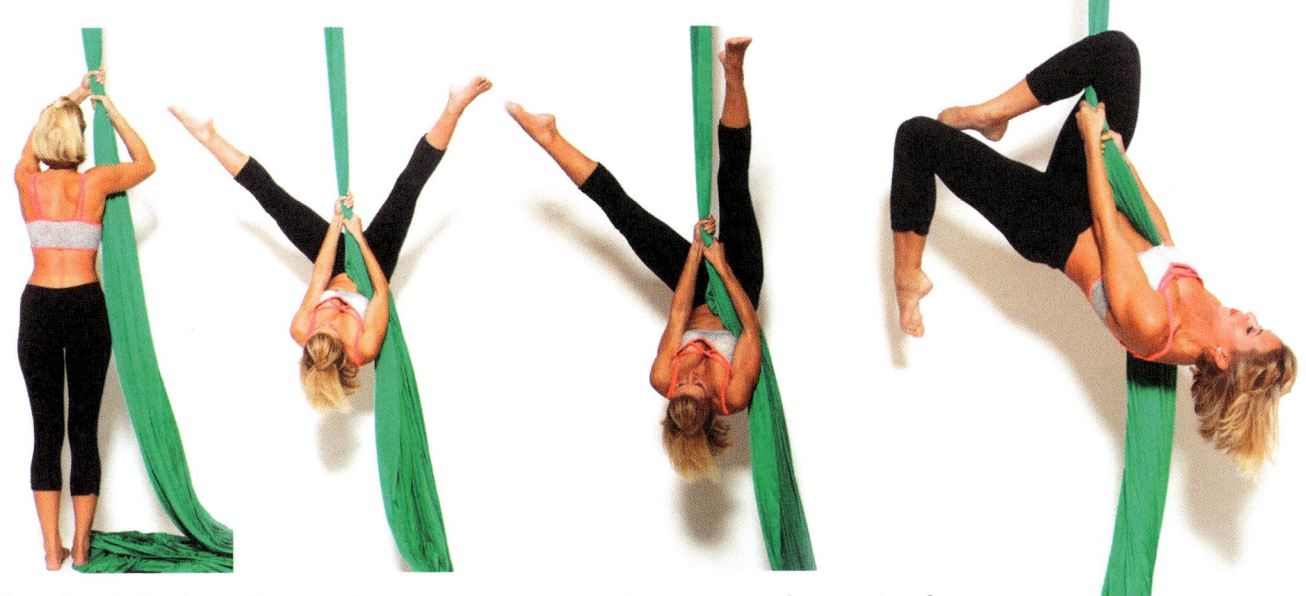

An inside leg hang is a precursor to many inverted poses...
The hang carries an equal amount of weight between
your hands and leg.

ENTRY
The inside leg is the leg closest to the fabric when standing at its side.
(If fabric is on the right then your right leg is your inside leg)

Reach both hands high above your head and pull your legs up into a wide straddle. Note how in the initial straddle the fabric is along the right side of the body and in between the legs.

Hook the knee (or the knee and ankle)
around the fabric.

SAFETY CONCERNS
The fabric must be along the side
of the body. . . many make the
mistake of straddling
up with the fabric in between the legs.

TECHNIQUES / TIPS
Keep your arms high above your head and a strong
grip.

PG 57

ANGEL

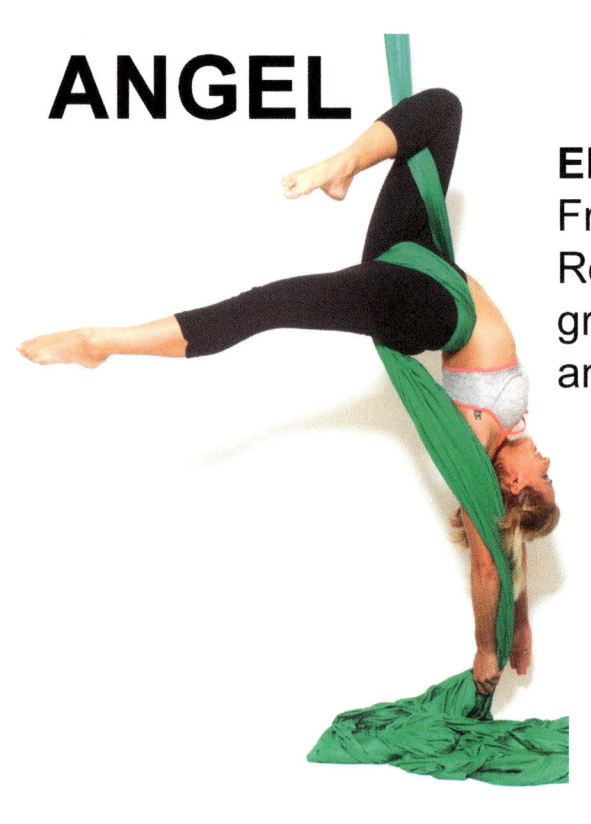

ENTRY
From an inside leg hang ...
Reach your free hand behind your back to grip the fabric. Bring the fabric to your front and wrap it over your free knee.

   (if your right leg is high then right hand holds on while left hand grabs the fabric to wrap over the knee)

Once you have wrapped the free piece over the free knee ... Hold onto that piece and settle into your pose.

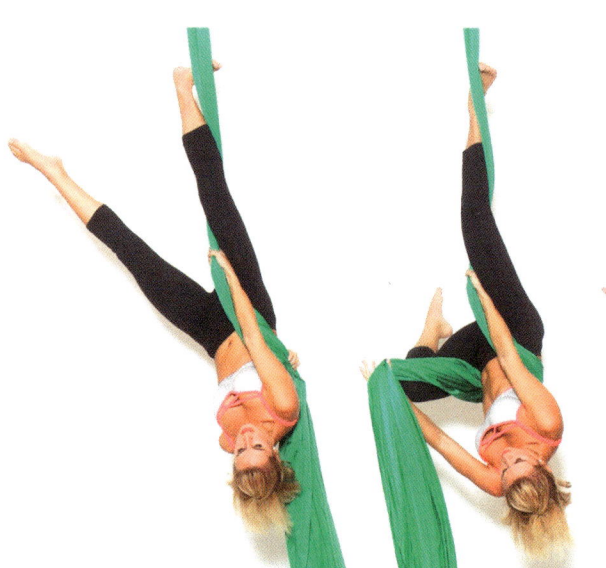

SAFETY CONCERNS
This requires alot of grip strength so be careful when attempting this on your own.

TIPS / TECHNIQUES
Some people feel wrapping the top foot in the silk helps with grip ... However some prefer to hook just the knee over and not wrap the toes.

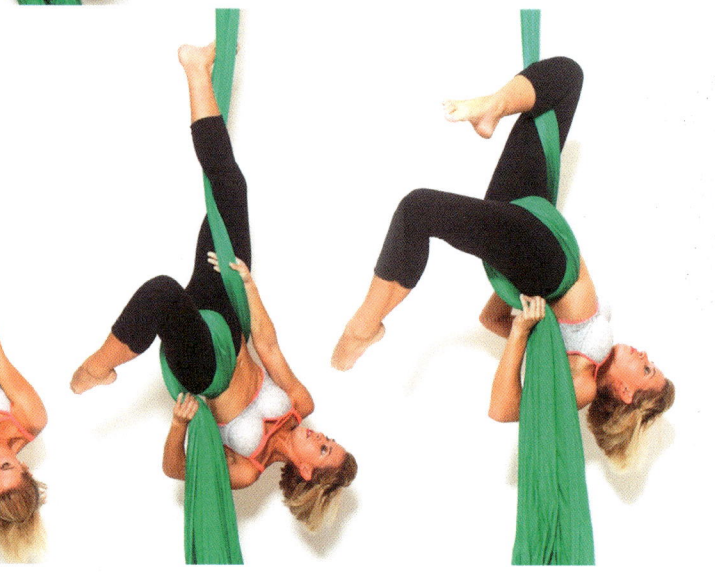

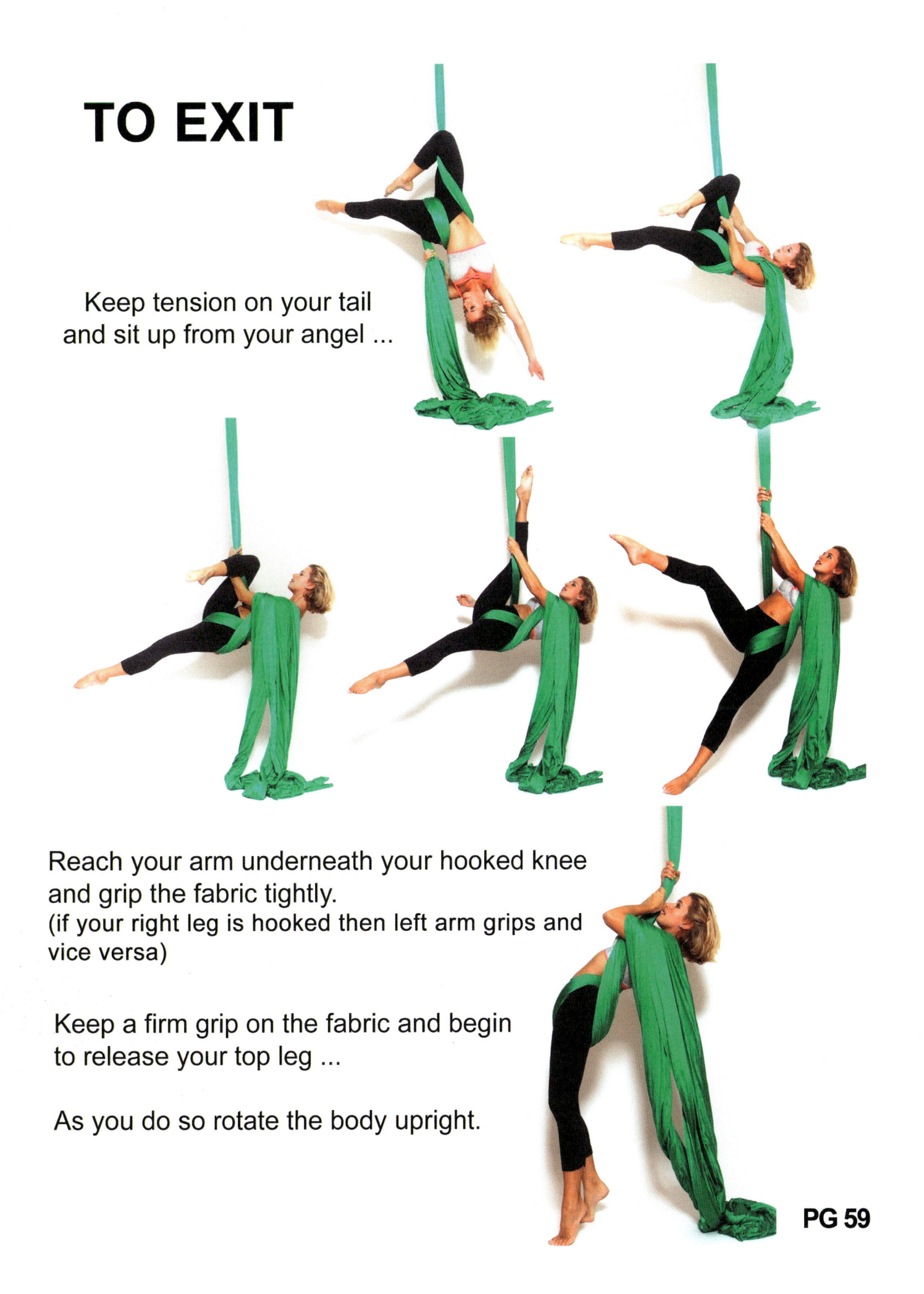

TO EXIT

Keep tension on your tail and sit up from your angel ...

Reach your arm underneath your hooked knee and grip the fabric tightly.
(if your right leg is hooked then left arm grips and vice versa)

Keep a firm grip on the fabric and begin to release your top leg ...

As you do so rotate the body upright.

PG 59

SCORPION

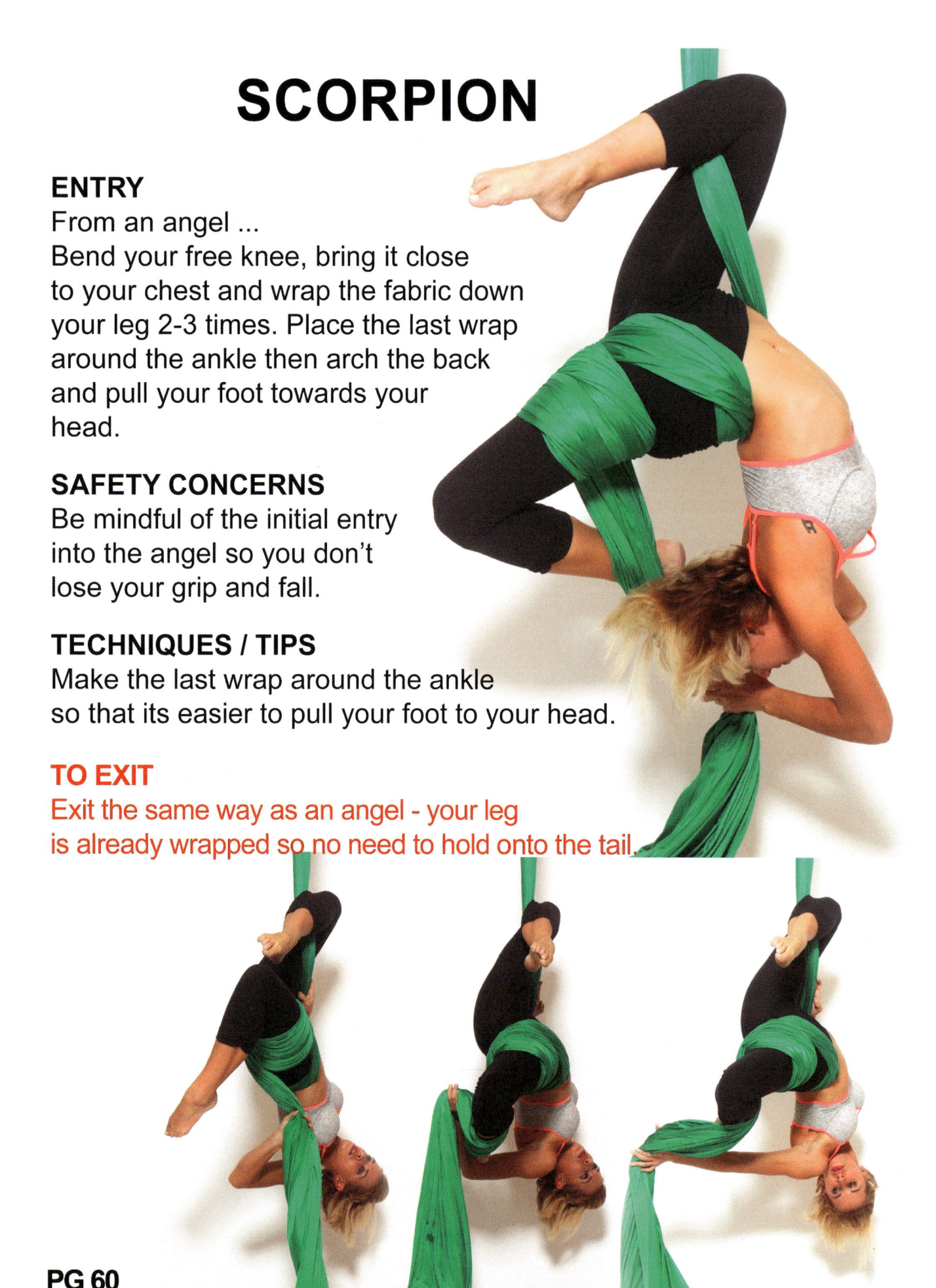

ENTRY
From an angel ...
Bend your free knee, bring it close to your chest and wrap the fabric down your leg 2-3 times. Place the last wrap around the ankle then arch the back and pull your foot towards your head.

SAFETY CONCERNS
Be mindful of the initial entry into the angel so you don't lose your grip and fall.

TECHNIQUES / TIPS
Make the last wrap around the ankle so that its easier to pull your foot to your head.

TO EXIT
Exit the same way as an angel - your leg is already wrapped so no need to hold onto the tail.

CRUCIFIX WRAP

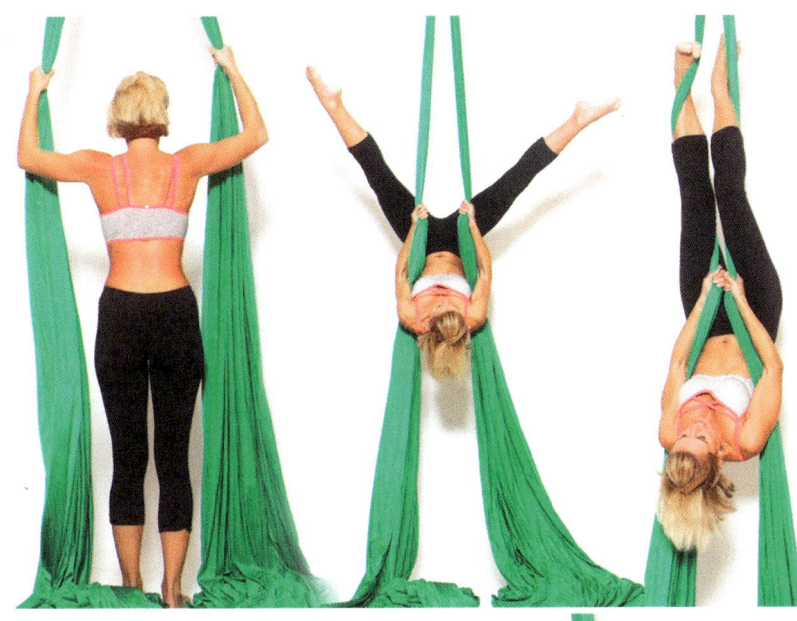

ENTRY

Split the fabric and stand in between the two pieces .. Pull yourself up into an inverted straddle and wrap your knees and toes into the fabric.

(note how in the initial straddle up the fabric runs along your inner thighs / pubic bone)

Do not lose grip of the fabric but slide your hands down the fabric to your lower back.

Cross the fabric behind your lower back and then bring the pieces to your front.

SAFETY CONCERNS

do not let go of the fabric pieces with your hands for you might slide down the fabric.

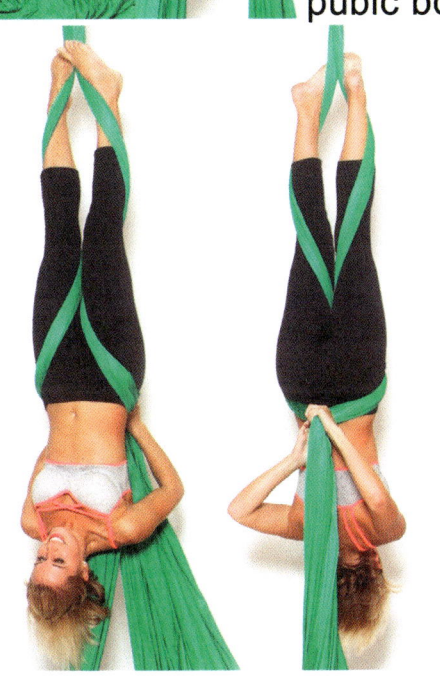

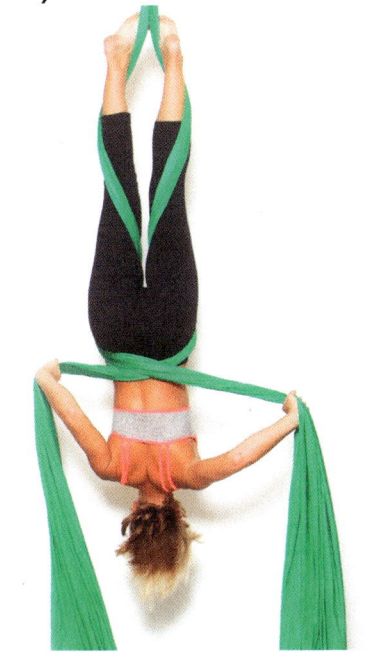

TECHNIQUES / TIPS

Use your toes to grip the fabric as much as possible.. squeezing the feet together or crossing one foot on top of the other helps with this.

Once you have the pieces crossed behind your back you can relax the wrap on your feet and even bend your knees.

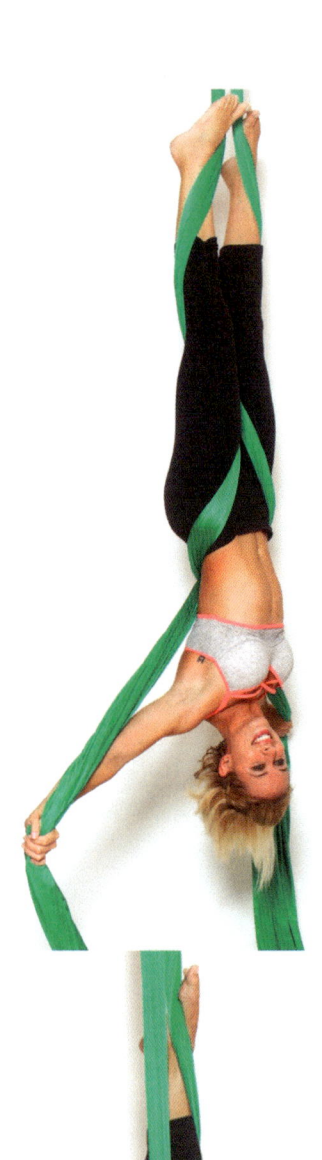

CRUCIFIX INTO PIGEON

ENTRY
From a crucifix wrap ...
Make sure to keep your fabric ends at your front.
Then take one leg completely out of the wrap
and extend it behind your body ...

SAFETY CONCERNS
Be sure to hold your fabric pieces in front of you.

As long as you maintain grip on your fabric pieces you are good to go. :)

TIPS / TECHNIQUES
Your top leg can bend or stay straight wrapped around the fabric.

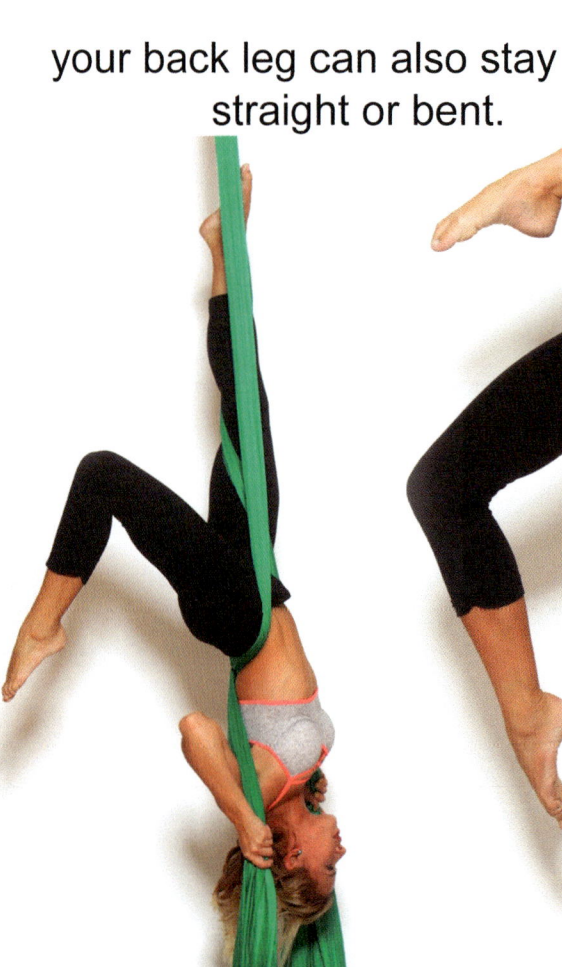

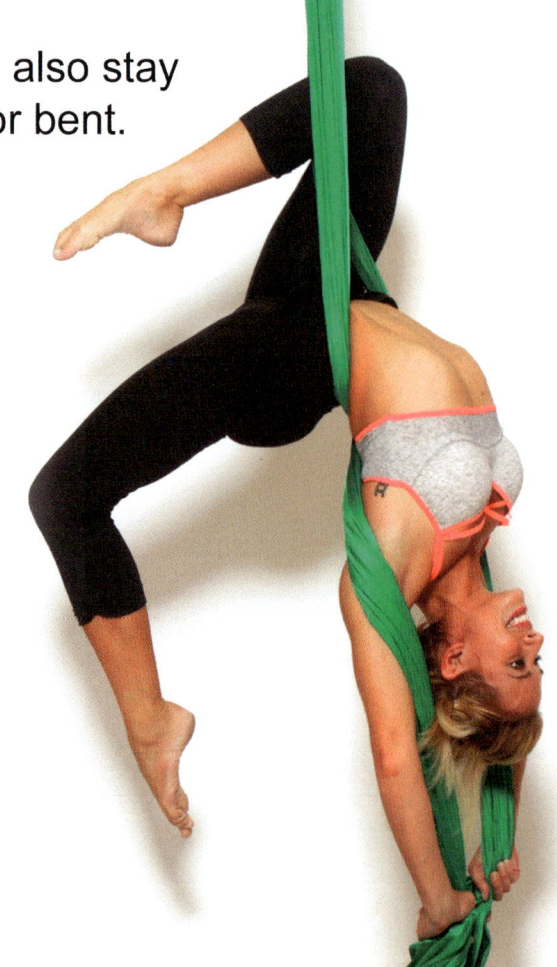

your back leg can also stay straight or bent.

CHAPTER 7
CONDITIONING EXERCISES

There are a multitude of ways to conditiion the
body using aerial silks ... But these happen to be
my three favorite for beginners ..
One for arms, legs, and core!

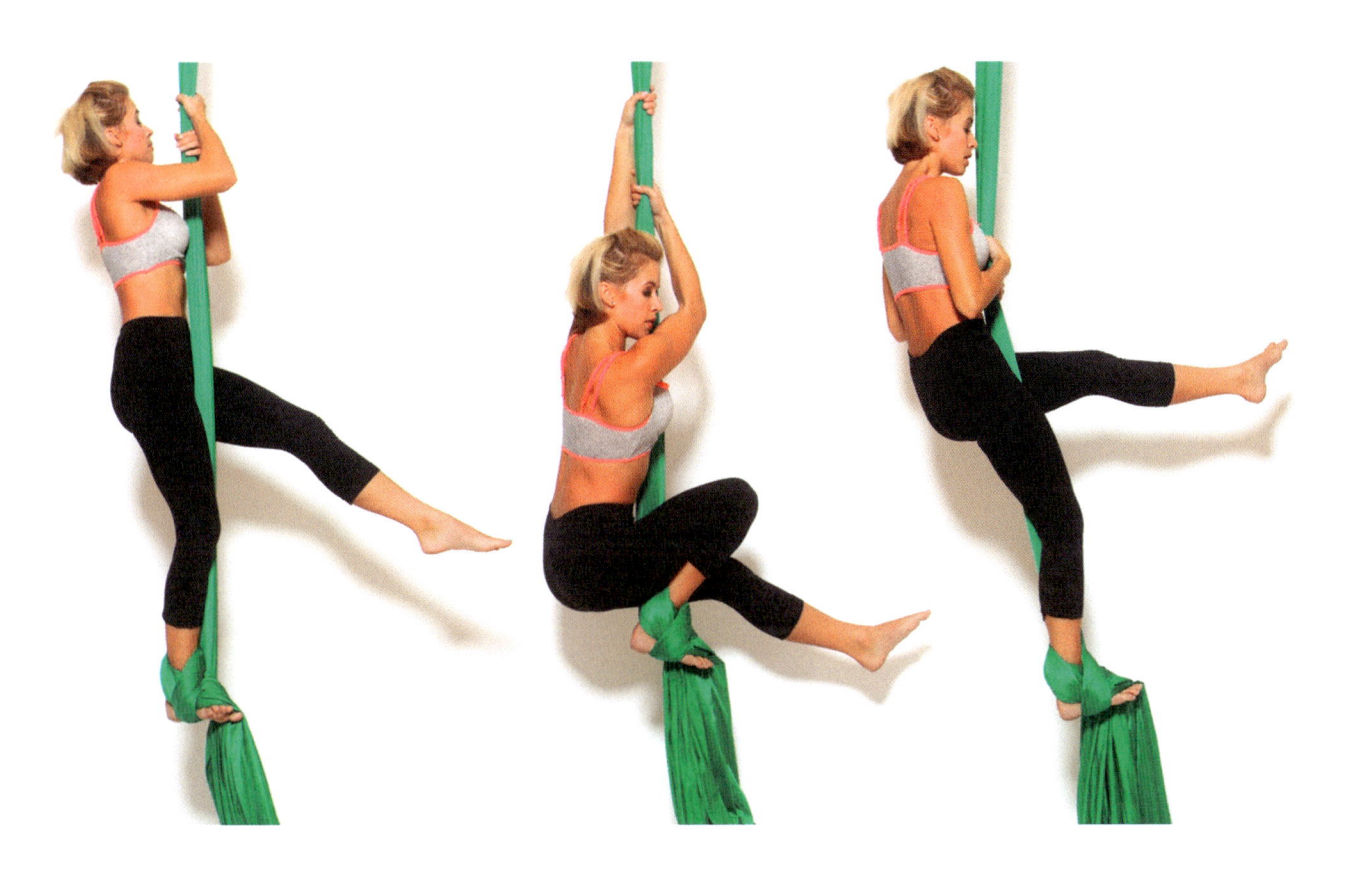

LEGS

Single leg squats:
From a single footlock ... Hold the fabric tightly and lower down into a squat and then raise back up.

If you are prone to knee problems then lean back as you go down so that your knee stays above your ankle instead of leaning forward over it.

CORE

Tuck ins:
Take a wrist wrap ...
pull yourself up into a pull up and hold yourself there.

Then lift your knees up and down as many times as you can.

If your arms are not strong enough to hold yourself up then come down between each tuck in.

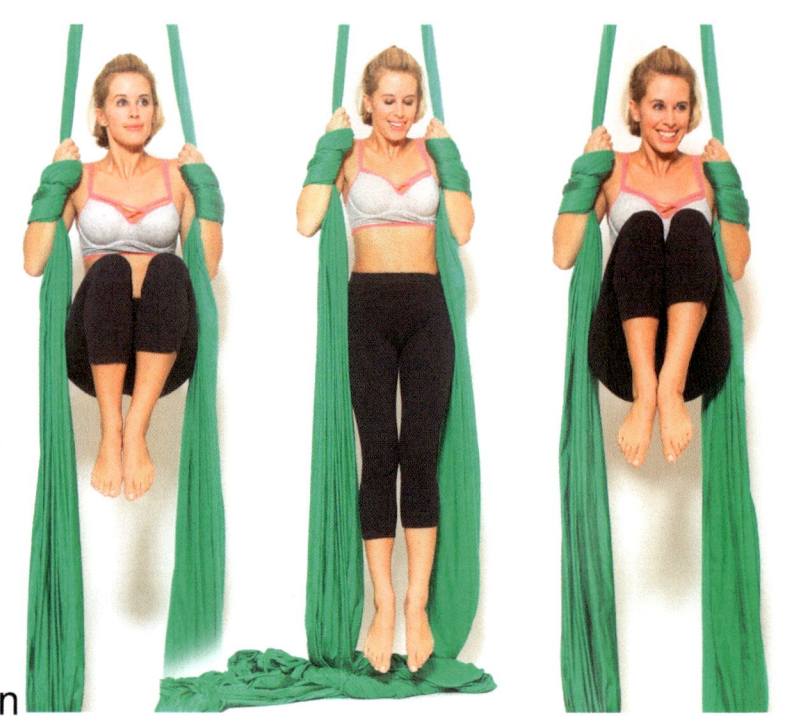

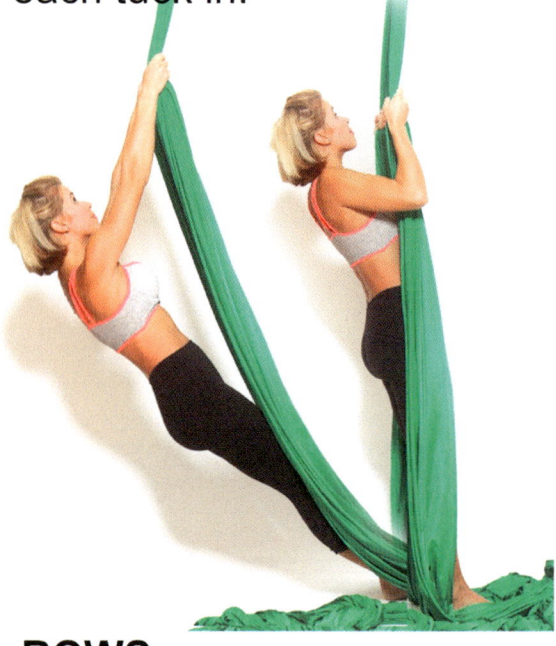

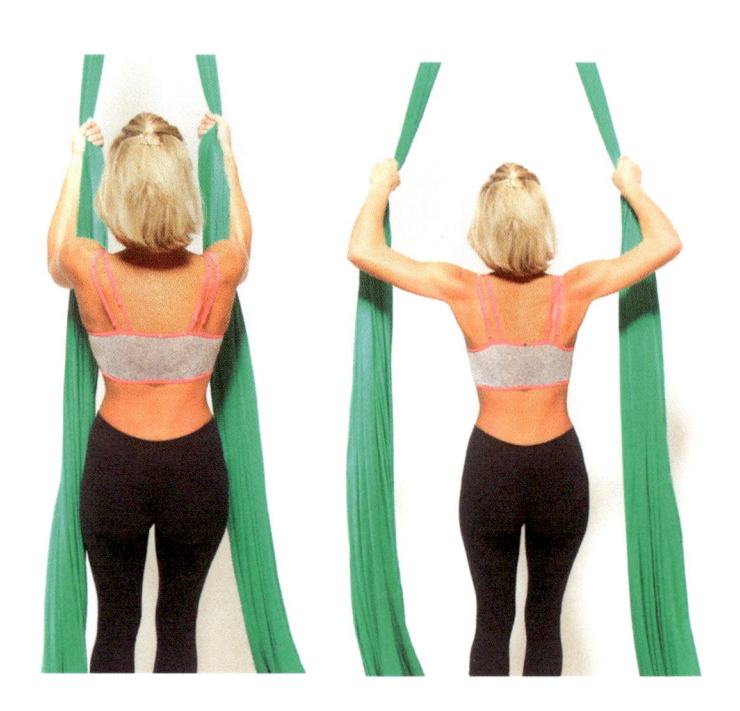

ROWS

Hold onto the fabric and lean back at an angle ... The lower your hands on the fabric the better / harder this will be ... Keep your body as straight as possible and pull your chest into the fabric and then lower back down.

Elbows wide for back ... Elbows in for triceps.

Remember to keep your body flat like a plank!

CHAPTER 8
INSPIRATION

"Aerial silks holds a special place in my heart and i hope that what i have shared has allowed you to fall in love with it too!

One of the things I love about this art is that there is much room to explore and use your imagination. Sometimes all you need to do is just get on the fabric and let your imagination flow!

The next few pages are poses performed by Sarasota Warrior students and I hope these will offer some inspiration to you along your aerial journey!"
<3 <3 <3

-Sarasota Warrior

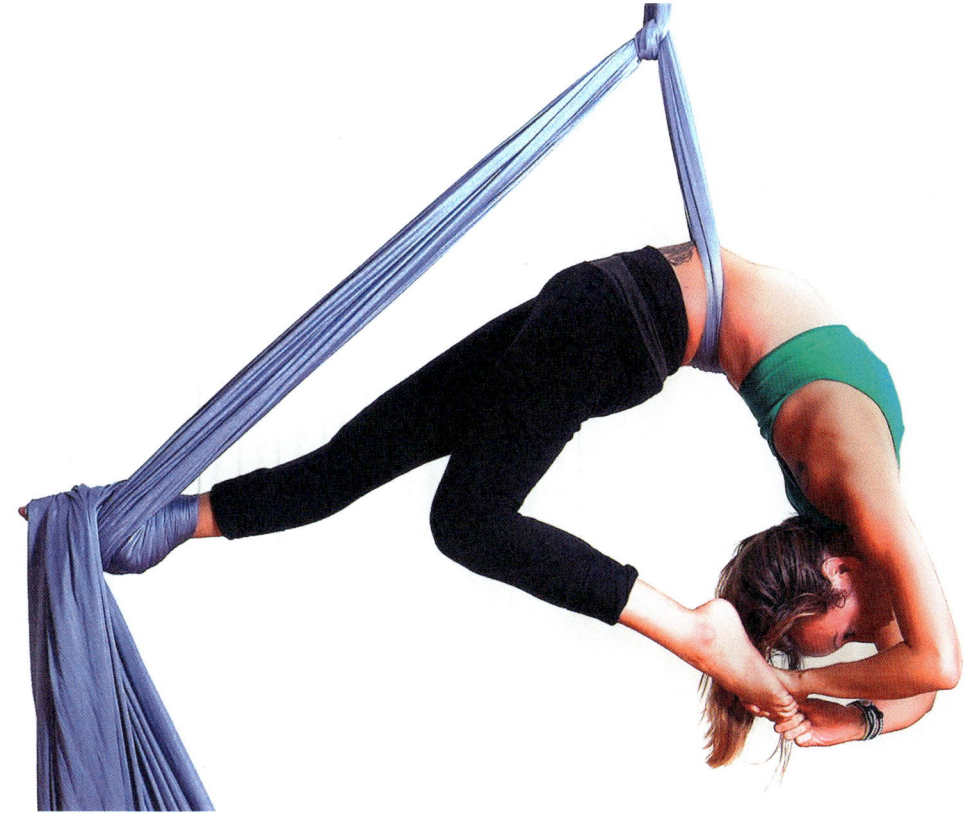

WRIST WRAPS

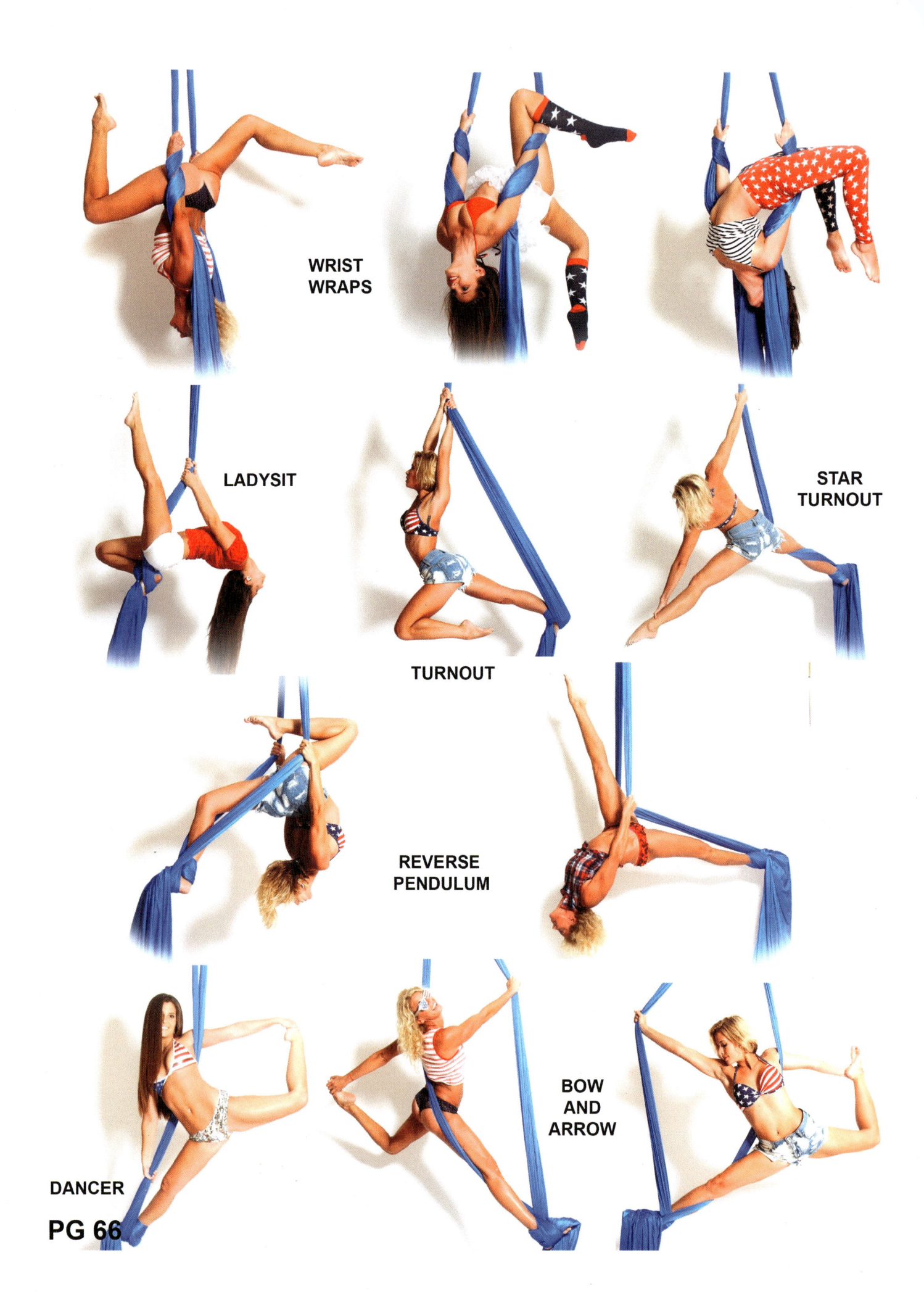

LADYSIT

TURNOUT

STAR TURNOUT

REVERSE PENDULUM

DANCER

BOW AND ARROW

PG 66

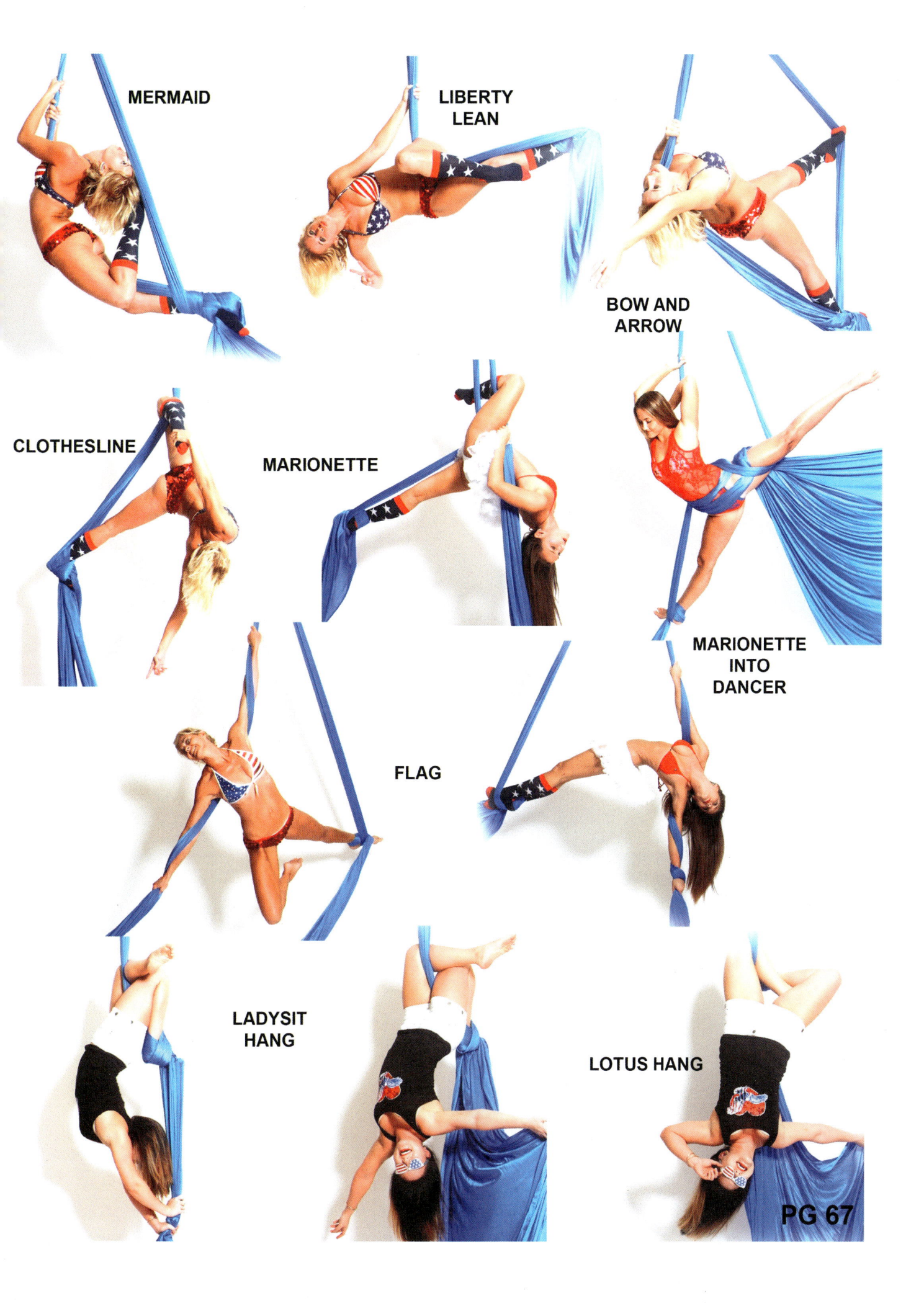

MERMAID

LIBERTY LEAN

BOW AND ARROW

CLOTHESLINE

MARIONETTE

MARIONETTE INTO DANCER

FLAG

LADYSIT HANG

LOTUS HANG

PG 67

CUPID SEAT

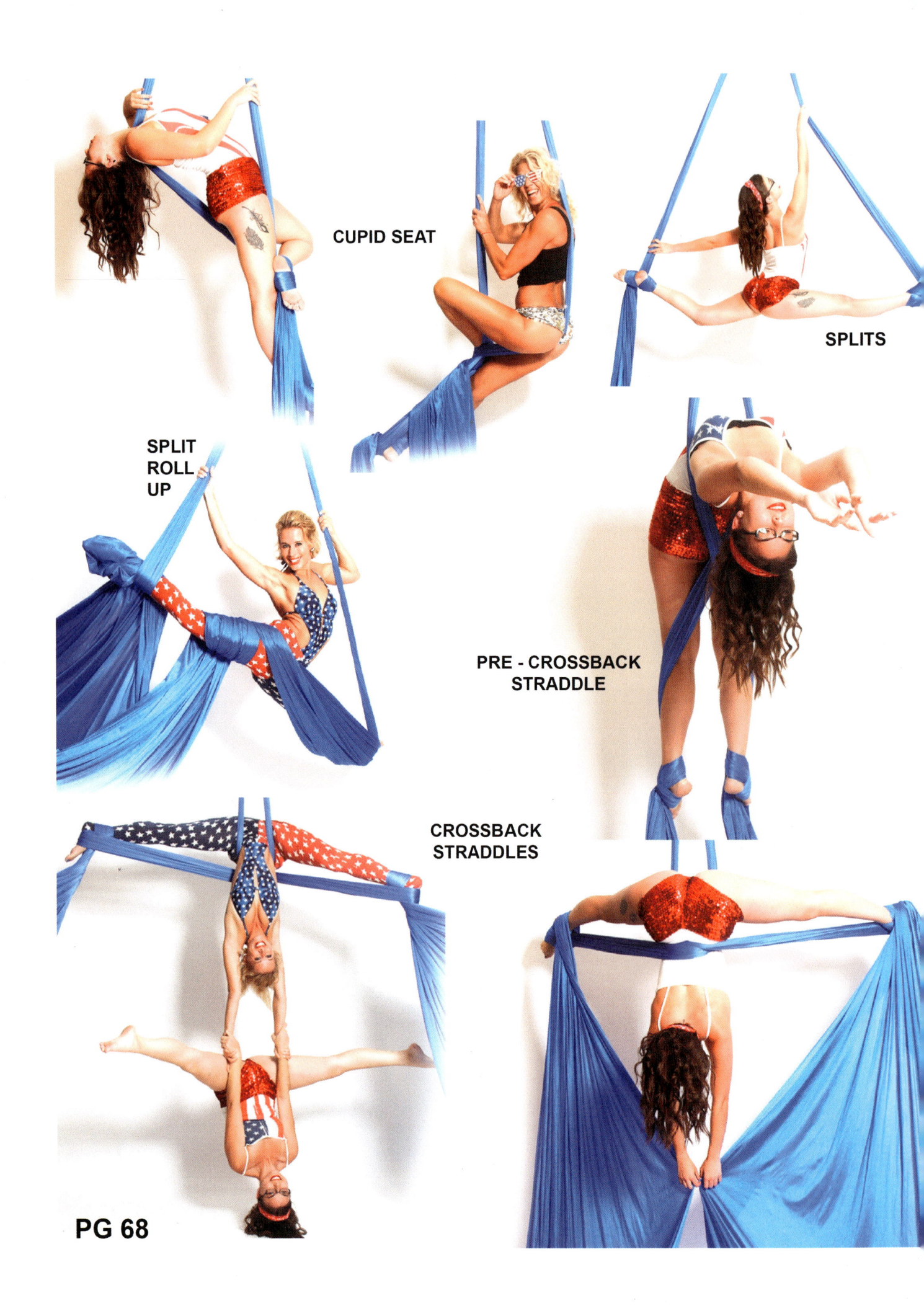

SPLITS

SPLIT ROLL UP

PRE - CROSSBACK STRADDLE

CROSSBACK STRADDLES

PG 68

ANGEL

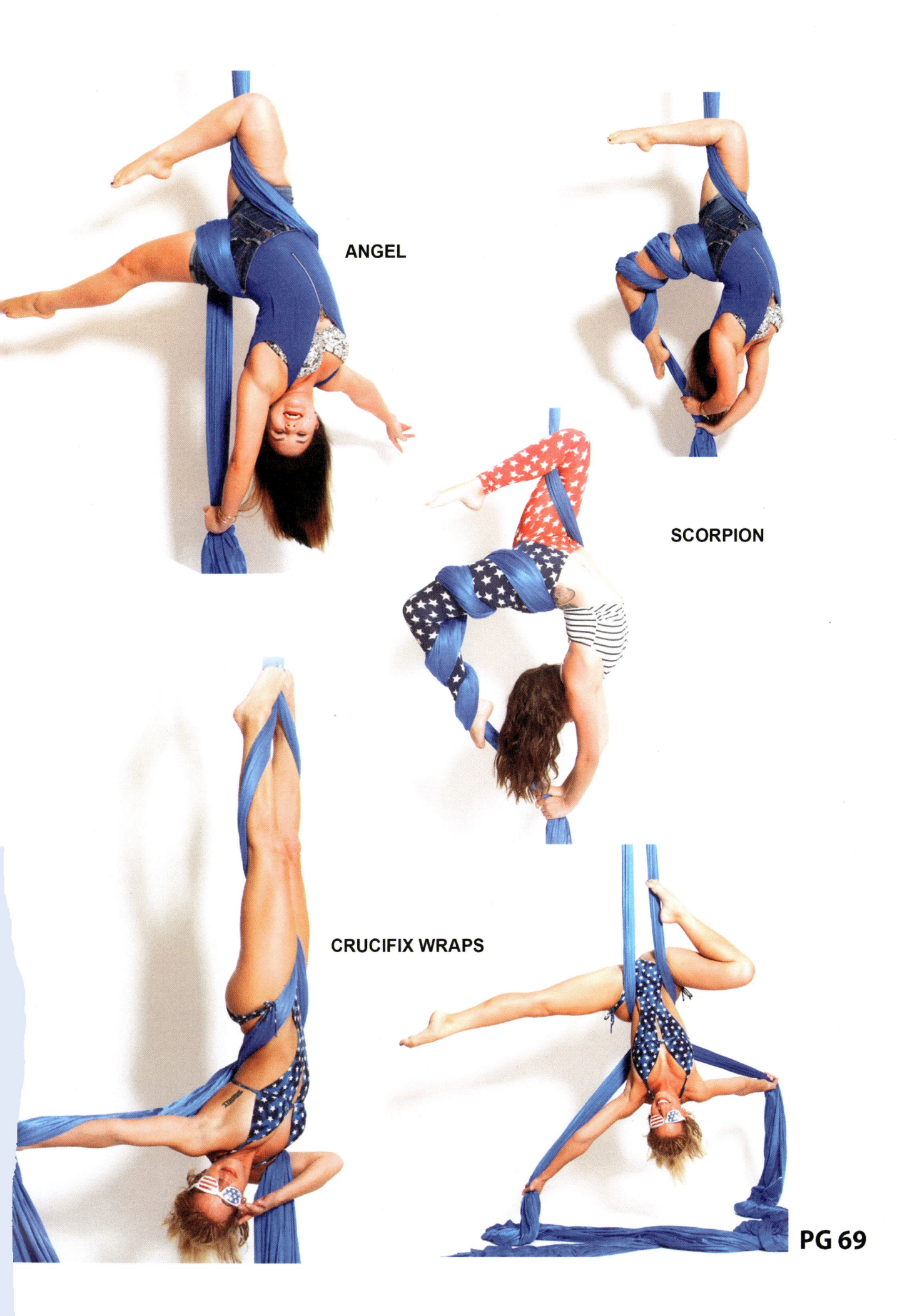

SCORPION

CRUCIFIX WRAPS

PG 69

Printed in Great Britain
by Amazon